Female Students and Cultures of Violence in Cities

"Julia Hall has edited a compelling volume on the reality and impact of violence in urban girls' lives at home, in their neighborhoods and communities, and at school. Against the assault of neoliberal ideology and policy, urban girls let readers inside the private and public spaces of their lives, where violence takes its toll but also meets with resiliency. Urban girls' stories of violence call on professional educators, students, and other stakeholders invested in girls' well-being to listen, heed, and take action to stem this dangerous tide so that girls the world over can lead healthier, more productive and empowered lives."

—*Amira Proweller, DePaul University, USA*

Feminism is positioned in neoliberalism as a throwback. In its place 'more relevant' forms of female empowerment are encouraged, such as personal responsibility and self-improvement. This volume explores what this type of 'liberation' means for females in areas of concentrated poverty and racial marginalization. With the absence of a social contract, girls in these violent conditions are more readily targets for sex trafficking, domestic abuse, disability silencing, homophobia, and overall corporal control. Exposure to violence has been shown to contribute to physical and mental health problems, a propensity for substance abuse, transience and homelessness, and, unsurprisingly, poor school attendance and performance. The modern girl has no broader, gender-oriented movement with which to engage. She has only herself, and comes to understand the self as a project to be worked on as a way to overcome problems. There seems no place to get away from any of this, even in school. Many educators have turned away from the issue of violence against females, seeing it as already addressed. In this book the reality of violence in the lives of schoolgirls in cities is put back on the map.

Julia Hall is Professor of Education Policy at D'Youville College, USA. In her research she considers the school and community experiences of youth who have been economically and culturally marginalized in cities in the context of a rapidly changing economy. She is also focused on gendered violence and female students. Her books include *Underprivileged School Children and the Assault on Dignity: Policy Challenges and Resistance, Canal Town Youth: Community Organization and the Development of Adolescent Identity*, and *Children's Human Rights and Public Schools in the United States*.

Routledge Studies in Education and Neoliberalism
Series editor Dave Hill, Anglia Ruskin University,
Chelmsford and Cambridge, England

Female Students and Cultures of Violence in Cities

Edited by Julia Hall

Routledge
Taylor & Francis Group

LONDON AND NEW YORK

First published 2015 by Routledge

2 Park Square, Milton Park, Abingdon, Oxon OX14 4RN
711 Third Avenue, New York, NY 10017, USA

*Routledge is an imprint of the Taylor & Francis Group,
an informa business*

First issued in paperback 2017

Library of Congress Cataloging-in-Publication Data
Female students and cultures of violence in cities / edited by Julia Hall.
     pages cm. — (Routledge studies in education and neoliberalism)
   Includes bibliographical references and index.
   1. Girls—Education—United States.   2. Girls—Abuse of—United
States.   3. Girls—Violence against—United States.   4. Girls—
Crimes against—United States.   5. Girls—United States—
Social conditions.   6. Students with social disabilities—United
States.   7. Violence in children—United States.   8. Violence in
adolescence—United States.   9. Education, Urban—Social aspects—United
States.   10. Urban violence—United States.   I. Hall, Julia.
   LC1481.F46 2015
   371.822—dc23   2015005885

ISBN: 978-0-415-86977-5 (hbk)
ISBN: 978-1-138-08494-0 (pbk)

Typeset in Sabon
by Apex CoVantage, LLC

Chapter 3, "Longitudinal Ethnography: Uncovering Domestic Abuse in
Low-Income Women's Lives" by Linda Burton, Diane Purvin, and Raymond
Garrett-Peters, appeared in *The Craft of Life Course Studies,* edited by
G. Elder Jr. & J. Z. Giele (2009).

Chapter 4, "Gender as the Next Top Model of Global Consumer-Citizenship,"
by Lindsay Palmer, appeared in *Genders Online,* Issue 51 (2010).

To Esther and Naomi

Contents

1 Capital and the Production of Classed and Racialized Females

Julia Hall

In the current stage of economic development, social freedoms have been relegated by those with power as an 'extra' or 'entitlement.' Whereas this has long been the historical reality among groups who have been dominated, now it is visible and felt by many who have been privileged. Missing in the culture is a sense of a larger, connective framework—something bigger than ourselves—in which we are linked to each other by our shared political commitments and commonality. Instead, people are left with only themselves to negotiate the struggle inherent in neoliberal productivity (Bauman, 2001). Countless are barely doing so, and a significant number in this category are girls and young women. This is the case particularly in communities characterized by economic and racial marginalization. While contestation is crosscutting, contemporary females are featured in this analysis as many of their concerns are assumed to have been addressed by past feminist movements (e.g., McRobbie, 2009, 2010). Women, however, continue to be victimized in evolving ways as an integral feature of capitalist relations. What this means for school age females living in neighborhoods of concentrated dispossession within cities is worth considering.

Over the past decade, my research on violence in the lives of girls in US urban locations chronicles ways in which neoliberalism produces gender (Hall, 2009, 2013, 2014; Hall & Weis, 2003). Much of this involves colonial class, race, and gender narrations/constructions. Co-produced by those with power within capitalist relations, such subject positions are devalued with particular exploitation among the intersections. The more diminished social and political importance is imposed upon females across cultures, the greater the increase of profitability to capital. In this sense, racialization refers to the process by which those with power ascribe an ethnic status of less value on others as a method of continued domination (Collins, 2008; Maldonado, 2009; Omi & Winant, 1994). Gender as a critical site of performativity (e.g., 'female,' 'femininity') is so well understood at this point in feminist theory it hardly needs explanation (McRobbie, 2010).

How the continuous devaluing of classed and racialized women translates on the ground for female students who have been racially or economically marginalized living in US cities is the subject of this book. It seems those who could change things have turned their attention to other things. With the destabilization of employment and the absence of a social contract, ever increasing numbers of girls are straining to negotiate their lives at home, in their larger surroundings, and in their schools as those spaces are becoming saturated with violence. What does a girl do when there is no place to get away from this, and even school is a danger zone? She may disengage from learning and this along with the danger itself likely has a negative impact on her future. Why have so many educators turned their attention away from this reality, seeing the issue as already addressed in prior decades? If it is acknowledged, why is there a tendency to categorize it as just another example of the generic, decontextualized, and depoliticized concept of 'bullying?'

Critical educators and policymakers who research the effects of neoliberalism on schooling have yet fully to focus on this specific issue. Thrown back on themselves to negotiate life in their neighborhoods and schools, as specifically explored in this volume, females who have been racially or economically marginalized may more readily become targets for sex trafficking, domestic abuse, disability silencing, and the military-prison-surveillance complex. Severely lacking places to critique, messages in media saturate with consumption narratives. Narrow definitions of beauty, such as in the reality show *America's Next Top Model*, contextualize meaning-making in competitive terms as young women engage in isolated projects of self-perfection.

Classed and racialized femininity has long been used by capital to discredit the state by perpetuating the concept of minimal worth. In an effort to divest the state from protective obligations and to divert resources towards private interest, it is coded the feminine 'other.' Efforts to undermine femininity are animated, for instance, in the image of the 'nanny state.' She is large, bloated, and wasteful. In keeping with this metaphor, public jobs in government and teaching are disparaged in terms of credibility and pay. In this discourse, the Western, masculine, and efficient private sector shakes the state from its stupor. It prescribes lean, profit-driven policy directed toward specific females and race groups with the intent of subjectivity modification and compliance across the life span. While impacting everyone, many such policies are focused on females who care for children and by extension the children themselves. Over the past few decades, examples of such legislation include the Personal Responsibility and Work Opportunity Reconciliation Act, The Kennedy-Kassenbaum Fighting Fraud and Waste in Medicare Act, the Senior Citizen's Freedom to Work Act, No Child Left Behind, school zero tolerance policies, and recent cuts to Medicaid and the Food Stamp Program. Resultantly, inside already disenfranchised communities, the evisceration of a social contract and the imposition of such policy demand new and compacted levels of flexibility, sublimation of emotion, and despair.

Classed and racialized femininity as a delegitimized set of subject positions is produced by capital in other ways as it extracts value. In neoliberal production regimes, the performative qualities of 'feminine' identity—traits such as flexibility, creativity, the ability to listen, and attentiveness—are increasingly valued as the worthy attributes of the female *and* male subject as worker, consumer, and entrepreneur (McRobbie, 2010, 2014). The economy today is intrinsically dependent on these elaborations. In fact, labor itself is becoming feminized: from the creative team member, to the mid-level manager, to the freelance professional, to the service worker. In the will to work, all must be flexible (Goodman, 2013; McRobbie, 2010).

Moreover, in maximizing labor output, neoliberalism continues to need gender to be intensely divided along lines of the colonial white and the 'other.' In such framings, 'feminine' traits such as flexibility, creativity, the ability to listen, and attention to detail are coded as the 'essentialized' white ideal. Capital casts the gender of females from groups who have been culturally dominated in naturalistic terms—as unwieldy, highly physical, hypersexual, and inattentive. These females require extreme 'correction' so 'their' gender can be steered towards more compressed forms of exploitation in increasing profit. History shows a main demand upon the labor of females from such groups has been the forced suppression of emotions. This has been an imposed requirement for some females from enslavement, to domestic service, to contemporary affective labor in day care centers and nursing homes (Collins, 2008). To a lesser extent, it has also been a necessity for women of low income in general and those in customer service positions. In interviews with white female flight attendants conducted by Arlene Hochschild (1983) in the restructuring 1980s, participants describe how they must suppress the self at all times. This includes suppressing feelings of anger, frustration, and exhaustion in order to inhabit the sustained cheerfulness of the role. Now firmly rooted in neoliberalism and its undermining of employment, flexibility and the sublimation of feelings are becoming the prized attributes of the subject across groups. Still, as in the past, the most condensed versions of this apply among females who are low income or from culturally marginalized groups.

Today, women from dominated groups often become the sole family breadwinner, thus further compressing labor pressures. Given the suppression of wages and rampant inflation since the 1970s, the imposition of crack on urban populations, and the extent of justice system regulatory functions, desolation for males from dominated groups has deepened (Alexander, 2012; Wacquant, 2009). Race and class profiling across institutions attempts to pre-write futures in limiting ways for many young men as fodder for the prison complex. For example, especially post 9/11, criminal history records can be accessed by the majority of employers (Alexander, 2012; MacLeod, 2009). Females today on the expanding margins continue to be disproportionately represented in minimum wage, unstable, caretaking capacities. These jobs include home health aides, nursing home aides, day care center attendants, housekeepers, cooks, and fast food workers. Such affective labor is physically and emotionally demanding and offers lack of control over time and space. With historically constricted access to jobs, networking opportunities, and education, there has been much less ability among families who have been culturally marginalized to pool resources to get through difficult times.

The exploitative labor of females from culturally dominated groups has historically worked to justify the undercutting of wages for all females (e.g., Williams, 1991). Moreover, as more women across groups have accessed higher education and middle class professions, Collins (2008) clarifies how this has been experienced differently for females from culturally dominated groups. As she explains, African American middle class women have not been spared from condensed labor. Such females who have reached middle class standing are more likely to work in shrinking government agencies. Collins describes how these jobs involve "the care of the personal needs of the destitute and the weak" (p. 72). These women are impossibly tasked with solving problems among deteriorating and underfunded systems and in overworked conditions. As Collins asserts, some African American women who are today part of the professional business class occupy positions that often resemble "corporate mammies." These females are there to clean up after everyone but are never really in charge. With the exception of those who are high earners, many women have several jobs and then compressed care taking at home. Increasingly divested of commonality, females must rely on themselves as individuals.

With the ascendency of neoliberalism, the collapse of the economy has resulted in the naturalization of precarious employment. It is ironic that while so much unstable and condensed work has historically been heaped on women from culturally dominated groups, the label of 'welfare cheat' has been applied as well. When it comes to an amalgam of structures that support single parenting, inflation, and low wage work, recent policy reform has resulted in new levels of devaluation for women and children who have been economically marginalized. The 1996 Personal Responsibility and Work Opportunity Reconciliation Act (i.e., welfare reform), for example, harkens to the colonial corralling of female bodies. Drawing on the same well-worn stereotypes as unfeminine, hypersexual, uncaring mothers, and welfare cheats, this policy is directed to all 'unworthy' women who have refused to be accountable in terms of work and sexuality. The legislation paternalizes, blames, and pointedly individualizes the experiences of women who find themselves impoverished. This policy effectively ended 61 years of federal assistance. As the primary caretakers of children and consequently the main qualifiers, it impacts women and children most. Due to structural racism, this acutely hits families from culturally dominated groups. With the reform, women and children now have a set time clock of benefits, between two and five years. Once that expires there is nothing else (Hays, 2003; Wacquant, 2009).

In the colonial tradition, strict corporal punishments await any who transgress the rules of this reform. In an effort to dissuade women from having children, mothers of newborns are required to work, and at all times they must provide evidence they are looking for a job or are employed. Most of the jobs 'found' by women are in unstable, inflexible, fast food type places. If unable to find a job, in order to receive assistance, women are assigned to unpaid, full time work in a state agency. Given the low benefit levels, substandard childcare is mostly the option. Any child born to a parent who is already receiving help is designated a 'capped child' and does not receive any assistance. If a mother unexpectedly has to stay home to take care of a sick child and must miss a day of work, this results in a sanction. The penalty for this specific infraction is the denial of all support for a month with the benefit time clock still ticking. This also punishes children whose rent, food, and heat are paid for by that withholding. Once the overarching time limit has expired, women and children are on their own. With no social provisions, survival depends on food banks, charitable organizations, and perhaps dependent relationships with abusive partners and the dangers of the underground economy (Hays, 2003; Wacquant, 2009).

As capital continues to produce classed and racialized gender, many are painfully feeling it, especially in communities in cities that have been most marginalized. As subjectivities afforded little importance among the larger culture, this violence is mostly ignored among those with power. The unnatural conditions of poverty and segregation are nerve-racking and relentless, and are themselves forms of intensity that create circumstances for further brutality. Whereas violence is known to cut across social class and race, females in areas of concentrated poverty across cultural groups are embroiled in it. With the disappearance of both employment and a social safety net, there are few opportunities to escape such conditions. Stressful family and community relationships can be characterized by isolation, conflict over lack of resources and conventional opportunities, and contestation over power imbalances—which may involve tensions around gender roles. Data indicate girls and women in such an atmosphere are exposed particularly to high rates of aggression, as both witnesses and as direct victims (Hall, 2009, 2013, 2014; Hall & Weis, 2003). This has been seen to encompass physical battery, sexual assault, harassment, and being the victim of a violent crime.

Classed and racialized gender as a constellation of discredited identity positions also shapes school policy, structure, and culture. In the momentary economy, public spaces such as schools, which represent physical and ideological sites from which to think, critique, and act, have been demolished altogether. Students are instead measured by ideologies, attitudes, and dispositions that align with market interests. This includes the tactic of division, in which all are recast as economic actors in an antagonistic struggle for survival. As reflective of wider cultural messages, in schools youth are positioned as unable to trust others and to see deep divisions among all (e.g., in curricular messages, in competition over resources, and in high stakes test scores). They are pitted against each other across gender, race, social class, and so forth, in an unwinnable struggle to come out on top. This form of schooling alienates and oppresses all students. However, given the colonial subtext of subjugation and relational silencing, this takes on new dimensions in decisive ways for females of low income, many of whom quietly live in fear.

In terms of gender divisions, today boys privileged by race and class are often viewed as situated on the losing end of feminism as the learning needs of girls have been 'over-accommodated' to their detriment (e.g., Brooks, 2012). In this competitive and discordant environment, claims of female violence and silencing, including sexual harassment, are often rationalized away as overblown. This simplified understanding of 'inequity' erases powerful linkages between gender, class, and race. It also implies too much has been done to 'help' girls. Whereas perhaps privileged white female students may have expanded opportunities in discrete subject areas, such as math and science, others have been left to fend for themselves. In the neoliberal social order, that which is 'classed,' 'raced,' and 'female' continues to have evolving and negligible social, cultural, and political value.

SITUATING THE INVESTIGATION

The cultures of violence presently experienced by female students in their communities, homes, and schools take form under the aegis of neoliberal expansion. As a global force, this process is reliant upon the strategy of accumulation by dispossession in which all areas of life the world over are subjugated to the uncompromising needs of the market (e.g., Harvey, 2005). In this system, human rights, environmental standards, worker safety measures, and public spaces, including the notion of the public good, have been forcibly dismantled by transnational corporations and their policy networks in the endless fixation with bringing what is outside within its bounds in subjugation. Steeped in the rationality of positivism, there are profound feminist and colonial underpinnings to this never-ending practice of targeting, isolating, cornering, dominating, controlling, and forcing of nature and culture into submission. Many of the most vicious outcomes of this actualize in the Southern Hemisphere, where the domination over the 'wild' feminine and 'primitive' 'other' has been the defining feature of colonial policy. Inhumane outcomes also take place in the North, with its history of state-sponsored land purges and forms of corporal control (Alexander, 2012; Bannerji, 1995; Collins, 2008; McClintock, 1995). Capital has produced racialized and gendered subject positions and plunged many groups into a history of violent devaluation in order to meet its needs.

Key to this collection is the operational culture of violence underlying capitalism. Brutality was experienced by populations from the earliest advancements of this system with the enclosure of common land. This resulted in mass starvation and a forced exodus of previously rural populations into urban centers where they were suddenly left to fend for themselves. Over time, this same narrative has continued, and has taken on new forms as a culture of hyper-individualism matures. Aggression is defined here as widely manifest—in structural, hegemonic, and personal ways (Collins, 2008; Rubin, 1976). It is historically expressed across all relations, driving the core impulse to dominate and control 'wild' and 'primitive' nature, and thus is innately raced and gendered. It is the central organizing feature of institutions and policies and takes on meaning within interpersonal interactions. Given the post-Fordist production terrain, violence is also cumulative, involving compounding, overlapping, and intersecting strands potentially experienced concomitantly from many sources. Such hostility, although intensifying for everyone, continues to be distributed unequally (Hall, 2014).

Cities are the geographical focus of this volume. Metropolitan areas today are an integral part of neoliberalism expressed at the supra and subnational level. With their scooped out public commitments, the future of any urban area is measured by its ability to compete globally despite disappearing employment and state retreat. Pauline Lipman (2011) demonstrates how 'urban renewal' initiatives are often manipulations by a city's political class to close schools and displace those who have been culturally dominated in an attempt to increase real estate values and credit and bond ratings. Likewise, the fear of economic instability jitters the nerves of those with relative privilege—including prime borrowers from the middle classes whose wealth is typically tied up in mutual funds and home ownership. Among this group, this correspondingly laces concern about their personal assets and of course the future of their children in terms of expanded competition. Inside cities, with school and housing reform targeting particular neighborhoods, those already marginalized are being further pushed into intense and concentrated areas of poverty and racial segregation. Policies that feature austerity, surveillance, workfare, prison-fare, and other punishment web thickly through these dispossessed streets (e.g., Means, 2013; Wacquant, 2009). Situated within these webs, girls and women experience relentless forms of harm. Boys and men also fare abysmally.

The tendency among those with privilege in the West to collapse biographies into a singular 'female experience' is rejected in this text (Mohanty, 1991; Spivak, 1988). This approach is taken here both conceptually and by presenting a plurality of voices in the chapters to come. There is as well a full rejection of race and class infused constructs such as 'urban education,' 'urban youth,' and 'urban schools.' In using such language, white middle class suburbs, schools, teachers, youth, and families are implied as the 'legitimate' communities, schools, and youth. Anything urban or rural is read as a racialized or class based pathology that must be controlled, neutralized, and contained (Steinberg, 2010). In fact, at its essence, present day privatization of the public sector—including schools—with their emphasis on targeting, submission, domination, and control, is a re-elaboration of the same colonial acts of repression and ferocity, including its physical and symbolic forms. In the colonial context, which includes major traditions of resistance, assertions of female violence and silencing have long been trivialized by those in power. As linked to this narrative, despite noteworthy resistance, present claims of violent school cultures and silencing expressed by females are often viewed as exaggerated or an already addressed relic of the past (e.g., Brooks, 2012; Pomerantz, Raby, & Stefanik, 2013).

VOLUME ORGANIZATION

With the obliterated social contract replaced by a culture of hyper-individualism, many are struggling. How this orders the lives of school age females across urban areas in the US is the focus of this text. All in this book represent voices that have been economically or racially marginalized. An extensive array of data gathering methods are utilized in capturing these narratives, such as ethnography, case studies, and policy analysis. In the first set of chapters, the focus is on growing up in neighborhoods and inside households. Next, attention is drawn to the structural and cultural space of schools. A pattern that strongly emerges is that females who have been marginalized are afforded such little value among the larger culture that abuse is overtly, deeply etched in their lives. Given its cumulative prevalence, it is also often seen by participants as 'normal.' Even more disturbing, time and again, many of the young women individualize their experiences and blame themselves for making what they come to see as their own poor choices.

Violence threads itself through communities in infinite ways. For example, sex trafficking, involving the entrapment, disbursement, and sale of humans, takes place on a global scale. Of 20.9 million sex trafficking victims, reportedly 1.5 million are in 'developed' economies. As children who have been economically disadvantaged are among the most vulnerable of all populations, it is no surprise that they are prime targets for traffickers. Using ethnographic interviews conducted in several cities in the Eastern US, Virginia Batchelor and Iliana Lane present the experiences of social workers and law enforcement professionals who are directly engaged in rescuing school age female sex trafficking victims. The voices of survivors, although now adults, are also included. As the authors assert, African American females of low income are prime targets for traffickers as they are often concentrated in under-resourced urban areas. These girls, therefore, are more easily accessed and less attention is paid by the larger culture if they disappear. Traffickers count on this.

Linda Burton, Diane Purvin, and Raymond Garrett-Peters expose the extent of physical and sexual abuse in the home lives of low-income females. They draw upon ethnographic data from the seminal *Welfare, Children, and Families: A Three-City Study*. This research was conducted in the aftermath of welfare reform, and the intent was to make sense of how the transformation was experienced by low-income women with children. Participants in this multi-year, mixed methods research were drawn from Boston, Chicago, and San Antonio. Looking back on the data and analyzing it through the lens of domestic abuse, the authors assert that physical and sexual assault runs rampant throughout these lives. Startling numbers of participants report abuse at the hands of mostly male partners, and by fathers and other adult males. This abuse is not isolated, and is sustained across time. It is clear with the destruction of social protections brought on by the reform that women and children are now forced to stay in these abusive situations.

Lindsay Palmer examines the representation of gender and consumption in the reality show *America's Next Top Model*. This media critique stands as an example of some of the larger cultural messages readily available to young women. Palmer focuses specifically on gender performance as it unfolds within urban spaces. The show's contestants must 'channel' the experience of female homelessness, using this classed and gendered experience as a mechanism through which to prove their malleability as fashion models. Their performances, however, are underwritten by the larger narratives they create for themselves on the show—are they from the US? Are they 'truly female?' Do they know how to look both wealthy and impoverished? The author also interrogates notions of homelessness and, by extension, the concept of 'home' in late capitalism, asking how *America's Next Top Model* links these ideas to changing articulations of gender in the early 21st century.

School age females in cities also experience structural and cultural forcefulness while in school. Using ethnographic data gathered from an alternative high school in Northern California, Aida Hurtado, Ruby Hernandez, and Craig Haney look at the fact that small but growing numbers of Latinas are attending alternative high schools. These are education sites designed for students who have exhibited truancy, substance abuse, and disruptive behaviors. They are predominantly populated by male youth from culturally dominated groups and are designed around a system of surveillance, punishment, and control. The predominance of young men in these settings results in a highly masculinized environment where verbal and physical aggression is not uncommon. The hyper-monitoring in these schools may result in Latina students reacting with compliance, thus undercutting the development of the self-efficacy necessary to succeed in education beyond high school. Findings reveal instances of gendered micro-aggressions that may lead to harmful outcomes for Latina students.

Linda Ware and Danielle Cowley consider institutionalized silences in schools—silences that do not teach youth with disabilities about sexuality as an integral aspect of social identity development. As they purport, conversations on disability, sexuality, and identity are long overdue among educators, who in their own preparation for teaching, may not have come to understand disability as a cultural construct. This results in infantilizing students with disabilities. When sexuality is considered in relation to such students, it is often understood as aggressive, violent, and something to be feared by the 'normal population.' Young people with disabilities then may be seen as dangerous. These are just a few examples of points of scrutiny in this book. The final chapters offer suggestions for change—glimmers of hope in an enclosed, painful, and stifling world.

As capital produces classed and racialized gender, females from the most marginalized areas in cities struggle to negotiate this violent reality. In terms of layers of silencing when it comes to females who have been marginalized, the lack of attention to these issues by the larger public, policy makers, feminists, and scholars is deafening. It seems most have moved on, viewing these issues as solved by the second and third waves of feminism, thereby further cementing the culture of silence (McRobbie, 2009, 2010). Inside these schools, such sexism and racism experienced by female students (and teachers), and the dismissal of this by the larger culture, is dialectically connected to the devaluing of public school teachers and schooling in general. This is argued to be the case, given the overall feminization of the profession and the reality that teachers work with growing numbers of students who have been impoverished and/or are from groups that have been culturally dominated (Carlson, 2002). As guided by colonial narrations and market logics, what is 'classed,' 'raced,' and 'feminine' must be vehemently undermined, controlled, and enclosed.

REFERENCES

Alexander, M. (2012). *The new Jim Crow: Mass incarceration in the age of color-blindness.* New York: The New Press.
Bannerji, H. (1995). *Thinking through: Essays on feminism, Marxism, and anti-racism.* Toronto: Women's Press.
Bauman, Z. (2001). *The individualized society.* New York: Polity.
Brooks, D. (2012, July 5). Honor code. *The New York Times.* Retrieved from http://www.nytimes.com/2012/07/06/opinion/honor-code.html
Carlson, D. (2002). *Leaving safe harbor: Toward a new progressivism in American education and public life.* New York: Routledge.
Collins, P. H. (2008). *Black feminist thought: Knowledge, consciousness, and the politics of empowerment.* New York: Routledge.
Goodman, R. (2013). *Gender work: Feminism after neoliberalism.* New York: Palgrave Macmillan.
Hall, J. (2009). It hurts to be a girl: Growing up poor, white, and female. In K. Ferraro (Ed.), *Women's lives.* (pp. 64–74). Allyn & Bacon: New York.
Hall, J. (Ed.). (2013). *Children's human rights and public schools in the United States.* New York: Sense Publishers.
Hall, J. (Ed.). (2014). *Underprivileged schoolchildren and the assault on dignity: Policy challenges and resistance.* New York: Routledge.
Hall, J., & Weis, L. (2003). Where the girls (and women) are. *American Journal of Community Psychology, 28*(5), 731–755.
Harvey, D. (2005). *The new imperialism.* London: Oxford University Press.
Hays, S. (2003). *Flat broke with children: Women in the age of welfare reform.* New York: Oxford University Press.

Hochschild, A. (1983). *The managed heart: The commercialization of human feeling.* Los Angeles: University of California Press.

Lipman, P. (2011). *The new political economy of urban education: Neoliberalism, race, and the right to the city.* New York: Routledge.

MacLeod, J. (2009). *Ain't no makin' it: Aspirations and attainment in a low income neighborhood.* New York: Westview Press.

Maldonado, M. (2009). 'It is in their nature to do menial labour:' The racialization of Latino/a workers' by agricultural employers. *Ethnic & Racial Studies, 32*(6), 1017–1036.

McClintock, A. (1995). *Imperial leather: Race, gender, and sexuality in the colonial conquest.* New York: Routledge.

McRobbie, A. (2009). *The aftermath of feminism: Gender culture and social change.* London: Sage Publications.

McRobbie, A. (2010). Reflections on feminism, immaterial labour and the post-Fordist regime. *New Formations, 17,* 60–76. doi: 10.3898/NEWF.70.04.2010

McRobbie, A. (2014). *Be creative: Making a living in the new culture industries.* London: Polity.

Means, A. (2013). *Schooling in the age of austerity: Urban education and the struggle for Democratic life.* New York: Palgrave Macmillan.

Mohanty, C. (1991). Under Western eyes: Feminist scholarship and colonial discourses. In C. Mohanty, A. Russo, & L. Torres (Eds.), *Third world women and the politics of feminism.* (pp. 51–80). Bloomington, IN: Indiana University Press.

Omi, M., & Winant, H. (1994). *Racial formation in the United States: From the 1060s to the 1980s.* New York: Routledge.

Pomerantz, S., Raby, R., & Stefanik, A. (2013). Girls run the world? Caught between sexism and postfeminism in school. *Gender & Society, 27*(2), 185–207.

Rubin, L. (1976). *Worlds of pain: Life in the working-class family.* New York: Basic Books.

Spivak, G. (1988). Can the subaltern speak? In C. Nelson & L. Grossberg (Eds.), *Marxism and the interpretation of culture* (pp. 271–313). New York: Macmillan Education.

Steinberg, S. (Ed.). (2010). *19 urban questions: Teaching in the city.* New York: Peter Lang.

Wacquant, L. (2009). *Punishing the poor: The neoliberal government of social insecurity.* London: Duke University Press.

Williams, P. (1991). *The alchemy of race and rights: Diary of a law professor.* Cambridge, MA: Harvard University Press.

2 Human Sex Trafficking in the City: Seeking Victims among Domestic Girls

Illana R. Lane and Virginia A. Batchelor

Human sex trafficking is often misunderstood as a bad 'choice' made by individuals who find themselves ensnared in this circumstance. The sale of humans as commodities generates tremendous profits for sex traffickers. The evolving global economy fuels and supports the emergence of this industry, which is often controlled by local, national, and international networks. In this web, women and children from low income areas are extremely vulnerable. Given the growing concentrations of poverty in the North, it is important to examine the existence of human sex trafficking and the targeting of girls in cities in these areas.

The United Nations (2000) Protocol to Prevent, Suppress, and Punish Trafficking in Persons, Especially Women and Children, Supplementing the UN Convention against Transnational Organized Crime, defines sex trafficking as:

> The recruitment, transportation, transfer, harboring or receipt of persons, by means of threat or use of force or other forms of coercion, of abduction, of fraud, of deception, of the abuse of power or of a position of vulnerability, or of the giving or receiving of payments or benefits to achieve the consent of a person having control over another person, for the purpose of exploitation. (p. 2)

Human sex traffickers control people for profit (National Conference of State Legislatures [NCSL], 2011; UNICEF, 2000). The purpose of sex trafficking is always exploitation. Therefore, it is important to understand that what is typically labelled as 'prostitution' is most often human sex trafficking. As noted by Kotrla (2010), some individuals are forced into sex due to their inability to obtain traditional employment. For those from impoverished backgrounds, prostitution may be the only way of addressing the socioeconomic deprivation that is their present reality. Prostitution in such cases is not a 'choice.' Regarding human sex trafficking, the individual is recruited by deception, forced by physical and emotional abuse, and transported and transferred from seller to buyers many times over (UN, 2000). Human sex trafficking is about power and control.

Some populations are more vulnerable to human sex traffickers. In the US, African American girls are prime targets of sex trafficking (Batchelor & Lane, 2015; Gordon, 2006; Tillet, 2010). Additionally, UNICEF (2000) identified the following groups in every part of the world as most vulnerable: those in poverty, members of culturally dominated groups, indigenous and migrant women, refugee women, those in situations of armed conflict, women in institutions and detention centers, women with disabilities, elderly women, and children. Whereas boys and certain adult males are also at risk (Batchelor & Lane, 2015), the emphasis in this analysis is on girls in the US as targets in urban neighborhoods characterized by a high concentration of poverty and racial segregation. Moreover, the trafficking of labor is indeed a growing crime and as such deserves significant attention.

Unprecedented numbers of African American girls disappear from their classrooms, communities, and churches in the US and become lost in this underground system of exploitation. They often remain uncounted because African American children are rarely considered high profile cases/victims among the larger culture and are considered runaways (Batchelor & Lane, 2015; Gordon, 2006; Tillet, 2010). Little attention in the mainstream media is focused upon the increasing numbers of African American girls being kidnapped and sold into sexual trafficking. Traffickers know this, which is why they often target marginalized urban areas. Therefore, it is important to be aware of how the influence of political and economic status, institutional racism, and media gravely undercut the human rights of women and girls.

METHODOLOGY

Data were obtained for this analysis from interviews with six women residing in cities in the Eastern US. The six women who participated in the study provided personal accounts about the world of human sex trafficking by offering invaluable information as social workers, law enforcement professionals, and former victims. As African American female academic researchers, we approached participants with sensitivity. As well, we included, as much as possible, the voices of those from a variety of cultures and backgrounds. Given the sensitive subject matter, a snowball sampling method was utilized. Due to this approach, the two survivor participants of sex trafficking (both African American) agreed to participate due to contact with the same social worker, also an African American. It is crucial to understand, however, that human sex trafficking victims come from all cultural backgrounds. Pseudonyms were assigned to each participant to protect her identity and to respect her privacy (Biernaci & Waldorf, 1981).

Participants include the following: 1) Faith, an African American social worker, is the lead forensic interviewer in human sex trafficking cases. Her career spans over 18 years. Presently, she works in a managerial position where she trains others on how to conduct interviews regarding sexual abuse; 2) Hope is a bilingual, Latina Deputy Sheriff with over 30 years of experience in law enforcement, breaking up human trafficking rings, and rescuing victims; 3) Keturah, an African American woman, is employed with the Department of Homeland Security. She is involved at a governmental level with the advisory council on faith based and neighborhood partnerships directed toward addressing the needs of trafficked victims; 4) Ruth is a white outreach director and social worker; 5) Esther, a survivor, is a founder of an organization that supports victims of sex trafficking; and 6) Naomi, a survivor, helps save other children and adults in her work as a prevention education coordinator. She is also a correction education coordinator and is presently studying law. Notably, the two participants who are survivors are now working as anti-human trafficking professionals and are providing services to rescue and support other victims.

CULTURE OF VIOLENCE

A culture of violence prevails in the US. The framework regarding social values that is imposed upon females and everyone is comprised of various western influences. Institutional practices and social norms that impact women's status within the political and economic sphere inherit gender ideals and influences from other capitalist cultures. Specifically, earlier settlers from England brought their capitalist, Judeo-Christian, patriarchal, Eurocentric ideologies and dispositions that legitimized the subjugation of females (SafeNetwork, 2008).

Institutionalized practices that supported a husband's legal right to beat his wife were not addressed until 1870 in the US courts. Domestic violence still remains a source of shame, and much goes unreported. Many women do not report out of fear of reprisal. Organized activism is still a necessity due to heightened violence toward women. The purpose of the 'Take Back the Night' marches and rape crisis centers that were formed by women in the 1970s is to bring about awareness of gendered violence, to provide programs and shelter to help victimized females, and to educate the public that violence is dysfunctional behavior (Jane Doe Inc. [JDI], 2014).

Cultural influences regarding sex are reflected in the media. Women and girls are continually exploited in movies and music videos. Girls are targeted to sell, for example, adult clothing, by capturing the eye of the consumer with situational and inappropriate adult poses. The fashion industry sends a message that exploitation of girls is acceptable. Ashley Mears (2012) perhaps says it best, 'A 16-year-old boy on the catwalk would be as rare a sighting as a 35-year-old woman' (para. 4). Media also glamorizes the connection between the pimp and prostitute through movies, music, and television, for example, with the song lyrics, 'You know it's hard out there for a pimp; when he tryin' to get this money for the rent' (Three 6 Mafia, 2005).

Along with other forms of gender violence, human sex trafficking is so pervasive a crime it is often immeasurable. Sex-trafficking victims are typically misidentified as criminals, leading to misinterpretations of their behavior as promiscuous and hypersexual. Instead of understanding those enmeshed in sex trafficking as being victimized, due to stereotypes of 'the happy hooker,' such individuals are often blamed for making poor choices. Girls in cities in areas of concentrated poverty and racial marginalization are prime targets (Batchelor & Lane, 2015). How much is a little girl worth? A young girl is sold over and over. Three girls can yield as much as $1500 a night or $10,500 tax free dollars in one week (Batchelor & Lane, 2013; MSBC, 2008). Children do not choose or have power over their bodies (Girl for Sale, 2010). To criminalize minors is to exploit their vulnerability and lend support to their traffickers.

DOMESTIC, URBAN, GIRLS: THE GOLD COINS

Human sex trafficking into and within the US occurs in every state (Finklea, Fernandes-Alcantara, & Siskin, 2011). According to Emery, Heffron, and Moore (2012), more than 100,000 minors become victims of sex trafficking annually. Of the confirmed sex trafficking cases, over 40% of sex trafficking victims are African Americans, with other victims comprised of those who are white and from other groups. Equally important, there is still a belief among some that sex trafficking is not as prevalent in the US as it is in other countries (US Department of State, 2013). Even with professionals in law enforcement and mental health and educational institutions involved (to an extent) in educating the community, strong misconceptions on this issue remain. This only creates opportunities for predators to recruit more unsuspecting individuals.

Human sex trafficking is one of the most lucrative businesses and is rapidly growing. Hope, a law enforcement professional, explains that domestic human sex trafficking is more profitable than the sale of weapons:

> It's the second largest money making crime in the world. The only thing that beats it out is drugs. Drugs are number one. Human trafficking is number two. Weapons is number three. Five years ago, weapons used to be number two. (personal interview)

She also found in her work that in some instances human traffickers are not male. She explained that in rare cases women who used to be victims become traffickers because of their knowledge of how the industry works. The sale of bodies is edging toward the number one profit industry because people are renewable commodities (Batchelor & Lane, 2015). However, as more cases of human sex trafficking are confirmed, child trafficking is identified as more profitable than drugs. Predators seek out children as they can be sold for higher prices because they are thought to have less chance of carrying an STD (Nexstar Broadcasting, 2013).

Even as awareness of human sex trafficking increases, traffickers are becoming savvier in order to retain and grow their enterprises. The government is working to place stiffer penalties and jail sentencing practices in place to deter traffickers. Although law enforcement professionals are becoming more informed, victims are still being arrested for prostitution and then bailed out of confinement by pimps who continue to exploit them. Naomi, a former victim, spoke to this theme:

> Most cops didn't understand the full-fledged policy until it was reauthorized in 2007 and 2008. I was arrested five times for prostitution at 17 and they [the cops] knew I was under control of him [the pimp], never did anything to even stop it, let my pimp bail me out of jail and come to court with me. When I met with my lawyer, the pimp was sitting in the room with me and my lawyer.

Human sex trafficking victims cut across race, class, and gender lines. Likewise, sex trafficking victims can be any age. Reportedly, the average age of victims ranges between 12 and 14 (Reichert & Sylwestrzak, 2013). Shaniya Davis was trafficked by her mother to settle a drug debt and died at age five (Netter, 2009; Saar, 2009; Tillet, 2010). Hope stated her oldest victim was 62 years old, whereas Faith, a social worker, revealed that she has worked with clients as young as 2 years of age. Faith elaborated on her answer to the question regarding the age of sex trafficking victims by saying:

> We do sexual assault and sexual abuse interviews for children as young as three, very rarely two. We try to get out of two, but occasionally, maybe about 1%, a two year old is squeezed in just for an attempt which is still unsuccessful. We start as early as three years old up to age 18; that is adolescents, for sexual assaults.

Domestic human sex trafficking is a very serious issue, and it is important to examine geographical landscapes and how location impacts prevalence. The trafficking of girls in urban areas of concentrated poverty and racial segregation is on the rise. With the lack of institutional resources and a safety net in such areas, these girls are easier to snatch and deceive. This makes the business end of trafficking these girls as profitable as the gold rush and victims as valuable as gold.

HUBS IN NORTH AMERICA

Fifteen sex trafficking hubs have been identified in the US. Each hub or region provides characteristics that allow the particular location to serve as a hot spot for the business of foreign and domestic traffickers. Of course, the reported numbers in an area reflect only those who have been rescued and documented. Real numbers of actual victims are imaginably much higher. For example, in 2010, 136 undocumented children in Phoenix, Arizona were arrested for 'engaging in prostitution' (Girl For Sale, 2010). In addition to the girls being prosecuted as criminals, a large number of individuals who cross over into the US from Mexico add to the high prevalence of sex trafficking in this state. Many of the girls are coerced into the commercial sex industry due to promises of employment (Girl for Sale, 2010).

Los Angeles and San Francisco are also top points of entry for foreign victims due to their major ports and airports. Eighty percent of human trafficking victims in San Francisco are women and girls. A total of 27% of human sex trafficking victims are under the age of 18, and 67% are under the age of 24. Portland, Oregon has also been identified as a hub as it is near a major highway that is popular for interstate trafficking. Its large number of teenage runaways and liberal views toward the sex industry place it as one of the top cities where child sex trafficking occurs. Portland ranks second in the nation because of the number of girls per week who come forward as victims of trafficking in addition to the numbers of child prostitutes rescued (Girl for Sale, 2010).

Chicago, Illinois is flagged as the fifth most sex-trafficked city in the US. To date, the state of Illinois has instituted laws that make human sex trafficking a criminal offense. Although these laws allow victims to sue their traffickers, shockingly, there are laws carrying harsher penalties if they are arrested and prosecuted for prostitution. Toledo, Ohio is also identified as one of the top cities in the nation for recruiting children into the sex trafficking industry. This is the case because it lies near the intersections of several major national highways, making it easy to transport girls into and out of the state (Girl for Sale, 2010).

In New York City, an estimated 3,500 underage girls are involved in the sex trade, and the average age of entry is 12 (Girl For Sale, 2010). Traffickers advertise girls and women as though they are *things*. These advertisements can be obtained through adult ads in borough community newspapers. According to Girl for Sale (2010), the ads generate up to 35% of the newspapers' revenue. In Atlanta, Georgia, approximately 500 underage girls are sexually trafficked each month, which means that an estimated 100 to 150 girls are 'raped for profit' each weekend. It was estimated that 10,000 victims, including underage girls, were believed to have been sold in sex trafficking during National Football League Super Bowl week in Miami (Girl for Sale, 2010).

Las Vegas, also referred to as Sin City, earns the distinction of becoming a center for human trafficking and sexual exploitation. Girls as young as 10 years old have routinely been found there in forced prostitution. Statistics from 1994 to 2007 indicate that 5,122 victims were rescued from domestic minor sex trafficking, and 400 victims were discovered in May 2007 (Girl for Sale, 2010; Polaris Project, 2010). Shared Hope International (2009), an organization that helps women and children in crisis, provides an estimation of 100 underage sex trafficking victims in the Baton Rouge, New Orleans area in 2006. This organization continues to keep the global community informed about the status of exploitive attacks on women and children and men.

Houston holds the unenviable status as one of the leading trafficking sites in the US. This city sits at the center of major highways between Los Angeles and Miami and between the US and Latin America. Its expansive international airport is a major port, and the city is so diverse that immigrants are able to disappear into neighborhoods that are minimally policed (Girl for Sale, 2010).

In 2013, the Polaris Project (2013) rated all 50 states including the District of Columbia with respect to how far laws have advanced in terms of victims' rights regarding human trafficking. This project began in 2011, and since its inception, 39 states have passed new laws to fight human sex trafficking. The Polaris Project members categorize the advances toward prosecuting traffickers rather than victims by four tiers, the fourth being the least effective. South Dakota (Tier 4) has not made the minimal effort, whereas Arizona, Colorado, Delaware, New Hampshire, North Dakota, and Utah (Tier 3) have made only a nominal effort to pass laws that will protect victims' rights. Eleven states were ranked in Tier 2, whereas thirty states were ranked in Tier 1.

Many cities in Canada are known as major transit and destination points for human trafficking, with Vancouver listed by the US State Department as an area of major concern. Tijuana, likewise, has a reputation as the 'Bangkok of Latin America' on account of its prolific sex industry. Mexico City's main international airport, Benito Juarez International Airport, is a global mainstay for traffickers. It is also the second busiest airport in the whole of Latin America. In addition to human sex trafficking, organ trafficking plagues Mexico City. Homeless children are picked up by unmarked ambulances, strapped onto gurneys, taken to hospitals, and drugged in order to traffic their organs. Children are treated like trash and left to die (Girl for Sale, 2010).

ROOT CAUSES

Economic deprivation has consistently been found to be a unifying factor among sex trafficking victims. An economic analysis of traffickers, victims, and the flow of funding for counter-human-sex-trafficking strategies is needed to understand this industry thoroughly. Chuang (2006) argues that human sex trafficking must be viewed within a broader framework that recognizes it as a global socioeconomic movement, transcending any single nation or state criminal justice solution. That is, understanding global economic deprivation patterns is essential in developing counter-human-sex-trafficking strategies. Equally important, intervention and prevention strategies must provide alternatives for victims and education for would-be victims.

Williamson et al. (2012) studied various social characteristics of domestic sex trafficking victims in five metropolitan cities in Ohio. Their findings indicate that out of 328 respondents, 115 of those surveyed were trafficked before age 18. From the total sample size, 12% were sold before the age of 12; 26% were sold between age 12 and 13; 30% were sold between 14 and 15; 34% were sold between age 15 and 17; and the average age was 13. By ethnicity, the two largest groups of those trafficked were non-Hispanic white at 26% and African American at 65%. These findings were similar to research presented by Emery et al. (2012). In that investigation, over 60% of those trafficked were African Americans. Those victimized before age 18 and remaining so through adulthood almost always came from impoverished backgrounds.

In their statistical report on human sex trafficking, Banks and Kyckelhahn (2011) found that males represented the highest number of human trafficking suspects. Interestingly, males involved in sex trafficking were white and black, whereas Hispanic males were more engaged in labor trafficking. Dank et al. (2014) examined what influenced pimps and traffickers to get involved in that industry. They discovered that traffickers grew up in communities where sex trafficking was normalized. Moreover, many were exposed to family experiences whereby the head of the household was a victim. Additional routes to the trafficking industry included influences from their neighborhood, such as gang connections, and early sex experiences with adults. According to Dank et al. (2014), pimps have a culture by which they take care of each other.

Keturah, a program specialist with the Department of Homeland Security Center for Faith Based and Neighborhood Partnerships, argues for the importance of funding appropriated for education, training, and long term services geared towards victims of human sex trafficking. Unfortunately, according to Keturah, there is a lack of understanding of the need for long term services for survivors. Government support falls short. Of the services that are provided, counter-trafficking strategies such as counseling, education, and living wage employment are scare. In this context, Keturah speaks about how faith based participation and state organizations can be pivotal in helping victims reclaim their lives:

> White Evangelicals have historically been on the forefront, not just the White Evangelical, but equally the Catholic Church, have really been stepping forth not just as it relates to training and education, but actually providing services for aftercare for those who have been victimized. They've done exceptionally well. I know by the grants they've been given by the federal government; that often is very telling. It is very telling for those who are getting continuous grants and funds to provide

services with the little money that there is, because there is not a lot of money. We know there is no money allocated for domestic. Very little I should say from the Department of Justice. The majority of the money is for those who are foreign nationals coming from the Department of Health and Human Services Office of Refugee Resettlement. In essence they (foreign nationals) have been at the forefront.

More funding must be designated for examining the cause and effect of human sex trafficking. The amount of money that traffickers make in the commercial sex industry as compared to traditional and legal forms of employment encourages the rapid growth of the business.

Not only are girls victimized by strangers, but they are endangered by members of their own families, which only heightens the physical, emotional, and spiritual trauma. Both Esther and Naomi were victimized by relatives. Both of these women say that as girls they felt unprotected by their mothers. Additionally, Esther was victimized by her stepfather, and this was not disrupted by her mother. Naomi was first victimized by a boyfriend of her mother and later by her father and brother. It can cut deep into the hearts of victims who are violated by the very people who are charged with keeping them safe.

Again, educating the community and making available more and improved services for victims is crucial. Survivors need opportunities to reclaim lives. This requires counseling, health services, higher education, and employment training. Keturah had this to say:

> Keep in mind there are those who will follow the money and there are those who want to get there before the money comes. It's sometimes difficult to weed out those who are serious and invested in this issue long term versus those who unfortunately follow money trails, and I think that is related to almost any issue. People tend to follow the issue du jour and it becomes their issue for the moment, and to me Human Trafficking is really what HIV/AIDS was 30 years ago.

Keturah hints that media could do a lot to educate and reinforce the urgency of disrupting domestic human sex trafficking. She believes the faith based community understands that it is a present trend and wants to do more.

EMPTY PROMISES AND BROKEN DREAMS

Human sex traffickers are scammers who are able to size up their victims' needs and offer them money, and sometimes promises of love and security. However, what the victim actually receives are broken dreams. Trafficking cases should clearly be recognized in those instances whereby underage children are arrested for prostitution. The very fact that those under 18 are picked up, charged, and treated as if they were consenting adults during the corrections process cries for a need for education and training (Polaris Project, 2014).

Vulnerable populations of domestic sex trafficking are highly represented by girls. Some of the victims are forced into the life by family members. Esther spoke to this theme. She explained that her stepfather was her trafficker while her mother aided. He broke down her sense of right and wrong, thus making her feel worthless. The physical, mental, and emotional abuse endured from his fists shaped a childhood of empty promises (i.e., parental love and safety) and broken dreams. After running away from her abusive home life, this further enhanced her vulnerability as she was swept deeper into the commercial sex industry by recruiters with, again, empty promises of a better life.

In domestic sex trafficking networks, there are always multiple players. Esther's mother's role was second in command or *bottom*. When it comes to the networked sex trafficking of females, the bottom, as explained by Williamson et al. (2012), is typically a woman. This person teaches victims how to meet quota and participates in doling out consequences if rules are broken. Much of the language of human sex trafficking is dehumanizing, referring to victims as animals (e.g., horses, stables). Other derogatory terms are, for example, 'bitches' and 'hoes.'

Recruiters, groomers, and watchers are very important to the trafficker or pimp. The recruiter, underage or adult men or women, is often someone the victim knows and trusts, or with whom the victim has gained trust through initial acts of 'kindness.' Groomers educate victims on how to conduct business. Finally, the watcher serves as an escort who makes certain the victim does not escape. Watchers have been known to accompany victims to and from court (Williamson et al., 2012). Naomi explained how difficult it is for victims to break free or even speak openly when 'perceived' opportunities are controlled by violent watchers and or pimps/traffickers who accompany the victim in court.

Naomi was sexually abused by her mother's drug dealer, beginning at the age of 6 and lasting until the age of 10. She lived with an aunt who later felt it was safe for her to return home to live with her mother. Unfortunately, that was not the case, so she moved in with her father who drank and a brother who sexually abused her. Her father demanded $900.00 a month for rent from her when she turned 15. This forced her out on the streets. She moved in with a group of girls who were 'employed' as prostitutes and strippers. To celebrate her 16th birthday, they took her to dinner and left her standing in what is referred to as a pimp circle outside the restaurant:

> I was surrounded by pimps in what they call a 'pimp circle.' They surround and harass you and intimidate you and try to get you to come with them. A car pulled up to me when I got out of the pimp circle. It was a 'nice guy,' or what I thought was a nice guy; offered me a place to stay and food to eat and everything else I didn't have. I gave him $40.

And it was a snowstorm so it was either sleep on a park bench in the snow, or go home with him. So, little did I know going home with him would mean I would become a 'trafficking victim.'

Naomi gave the 'nice guy' her last $40 only to become his property. Many girls are wooed and tricked by promises of undying love. A convicted pimp testified, according to Green (2009), a reporter for the *Seattle Times*, that an insecure girl can be coerced into selling herself for a dream of a promising future that he would provide. However Naomi, a naive young girl, was duped by other girls she knew and trusted. What she thought was payment for a warm night at a hotel became endless nights of terror.

Freedom is not as easy to gain when one has endured emotional and physical abuse. Human sex trafficking networks are comprised of criminals who work strategically to maintain strongholds upon their victims by any means necessary. Victims of human sex trafficking are typically held hostage physically, mentally, and emotionally. Although, as Naomi explained, in her case, 'a trafficker usually does not want his girls to use drugs because it lowers the property value.' She further conveys that she fought until she gave in. She described her experience:

> I had a potato peeler put to my face; skin peeled off my face, he ate it as a way of marking me his property. I have scars on my stomach and back because I tried to fight back; I've had several teeth broken, several ribs broken, my jaw broken because I tried to fight back. Then you stop fighting.

For Esther, the threat of hurting her younger sisters was the stronghold that maintained control over her decision to fight, flee, or surrender to her perpetrator:

> When I was 7 years old, I knew that I was going to become a protector of girls and women. That's when my 23-year-old cousin decided that he should sodomize and rape me in the basement of my grandparents' home, and I had to allow him to do those things to me, things that I cannot even explain to you today. So that he would not do it to my 3- and 4-year-old sisters, because that was the threat he hung over my head. If you don't come when I call you I will take your sisters. So in order to protect them, I would have to avail my body and my spirit to him for his perversion and his pleasure. So I became a protector at 7 of girls; and, I've been protecting women and girls all of my life.

Naomi and Esther explain that they ultimately became victimized in their lives by several different traffickers. Esther tells that this resulted in her becoming a fighter when she got older:

> Like a man, I knew that I could fight people and I would fight all who would try to do harm to me. I would tell other women 'you can fight

back.' They would tell me, 'you just a fool. He's goin' kill you.' (Esther responding to other victims: 'He ain't goin' kill me.') I just didn't understand how they didn't want to fight. I thought we were supposed to fight for our lives. That was in the literal sense, as well as figuratively. But they didn't want to fight and maybe they were smarter than me. Maybe they understood fighting would get them closer to death sooner, and I didn't know that part.

Naomi spoke briefly about the Stockholm syndrome as an additional context as to why victims do not always run away when perceived to have a chance. Victims undergo so many traumas that it is comparable to soldiers who experience shellshock and become indebted to their abductors for sparing their lives rather than to their rescuers for actually saving their lives (Klein, 2013). Education is essential for people who can make a difference for victims of human sex trafficking and for potential victims to facilitate change toward preventing further growth of this industry.

PREVENTION AND INTERVENTION

Education and training for interveners, prospective victims, and victims is essential on the ground floor. Williamson et al. (2012) developed an assessment and intervention tool to assist in identifying victims of domestic human sex trafficking. Simply put, whereas interveners may not always have positions on policy-making levels, they are on the forefront as principals, teachers, students, mental health professionals, law enforcement professionals, health professionals, faith based professionals, church members, family members, and friends.

Ruth, a social worker, is employed as an outreach director for an anti-human-trafficking network. She expresses how her work includes education outreach with a focus on gender-based violence. She explains that one of the goals is to make sure that people are aware of this and other trusted organizations in the community:

> One of the goals for the team is to pretty much saturate the city and make sure everybody has at least heard of 'the organization' so that we can start to build a positive reputation and get into as many schools and groups that work with youth as possible.

The organization has partnered with others in the US to enlarge their anti-trafficking scope. It is imperative that anti-trafficking networks grow larger than human sex trafficking networks.

Faith provides training for personnel in the Department of Juvenile Services to make sure that children who have been arrested for prostitution are not categorized as criminals, but are re-categorized as victims. The training she provides prepares individuals to recognize victims, hopefully before they are arrested and dragged into court. Faith describes some of the understanding she tries to impart:

> What is domestic sexual trafficking? What does it look like? What are the risk factors? What are the behaviors? What is *pimp culture*? What is *trauma bonding*? What is the reason that a 16-year -old juvenile has been involved in the lifestyle or the game for so many years, for 4 or 5 years? How are they continuing to stay with this person who has brutalized them, who has sexually traumatized them, who has emotionally caused them to feel like they are less than dirt, who has literally just made them feel unworthy, unvalued, not appreciating them and stomping all over their integrity?

According to Faith, it is important to teach about, for example, trauma bonding, to promote an understanding of why victims may be apt to remain in unsafe relationships. Additionally, a deeper understanding of trauma bonding serves to dispel stereotypes that portray victims as non-compliant in terms of their rescue.

Keturah's work at the policy-making level extends to her personal vocation of working closely with non-government organizations and the faith based community. As she explains, human sex trafficking is so daunting that everyday people are unsure of how they can make a difference. She stresses the importance of people helping to open the doors of churches to provide safe places for young people:

> Another thing in the black community I have seen done well is having mentors within the church. We can't underestimate the need for young persons to have mentors who can support them. Sometimes mom and dad are not always available. If they are available, great! If they're not there to have that adult supervision, someone who will be present for them is an incredible opportunity to intervene on a young person's behalf, but also prevent the opportunity of them engaging in any type of risk taking behavior. And for me, I think these are some baseline things that the church can do.

Hope's work impacts the criminal justice system. She continues to educate and provide training for law enforcement professionals, such as police officers, sheriffs, attorneys, and judges. She advocates that such training should become mandatory. In addition to working with trafficking victims and informing the community about human sex trafficking through the media, she has formed a foundation along with two public school teachers.

Faith continues to conduct training for her staff. She works closely with victims. She attributes her success with clients to working alongside mental health professionals who were once victims:

> And when they see that somebody who looks like them, who knows them, who's been in their shoes, who's operated the same way that

they're operating now, and is no longer operating that way. They're [counselor] operating in a place of strength, a place of power, a place of assurance, a place of acknowledgement, of worth and self-assertiveness. Then they [victim] can see, oh, if they got out, then, I can get out too! So I think it's very beneficial for survivors who are professionals, to work alongside professionals who are not survivors of sexual trafficking.

Naomi, a survivor, works alongside professionals who are not survivors. She also works with law enforcement professionals. She helps them to assist victims with care. As a survivor, advocate, and media relations expert, she also instructs teachers on how to educate students about commercial sex-ploitation and human trafficking. She says this is part of her healing.

Esther founded a non-profit organization that provides training, employ-ment, and counseling for victims that extends way beyond the initial rescue. She works with the victims to help them reclaim their lives:

> Being able to go into a college situation and not get a background check so that everybody knows who she was. I have to build those systems for them to have a life because rescue is not a singular act in my business; at least not the way I approach it because it's not merely enough for me to get them off the street or to accept them from a law enforcement agency or a parent or a judge. I have to now make sure that I can give them an education; and that's what I do at my learning center. I have to make sure that I can also have them employable and not at minimum wage, a living wage. Thirdly, I have to make sure that if they don't want to go to college or technical school, I have to help them develop their skill-set so that they can be entrepreneurs. That's the kind of work that I do in a center in Atlanta. I have memorandums of understanding with six colleges and finishing up with a seventh one so that my young girls and women can enter college and we can waive fees and we can waive taxes and we can waive background checks that have been mandated by the State of Georgia so my girls will not be targeted and people will not know their past, which will make them flee from the college.

It is important, as Esther has expressed, to understand that it is not enough to identify and rescue victims just to leave them without a future. Whereas these survivors are doing so much to try to educate others and help victims become survivors, the state is failing in its obligations to protect people. Moreover, her analysis is true for all 50 states.

CONCLUSION

Large numbers of African American girls who disappear from their class-rooms, communities, and churches become victims of human sex traffick-ers. They often remain missing, as African American children for the most part do not receive the same mainstream media attention as those of the dominant culture (Batchelor & Lane, 2015; Gordon, 2006; Tillet, 2010). Traffickers are aware of this, which is why racially and economically marginalized urban areas are targeted for finding victims. The two participants who are survivors of sex trafficking in this investigation now work to provide education for the community, the judicial system, schools, and the medical profession. They both say they can only now help others because they were helped. Yet in the current economy, the social safety net has been fully under attack. This is severely limiting the ability to combat human trafficking on all levels. For every survivor there are thousands, if not hundreds of thousands, of victims who remain so, and many of them are children.

The lyrics to the song *Olivia, Lost and Turned Out*, written by Anthony (1978) and sung by The Whispers, is an illustration of how a hypnotic melody can displace an urgent message, even while the listener sings the words of despair. The smooth sounds of the song are comparable to the trafficker's empty promises. Olivia, the victim, got distracted and then abducted by a predator on her way to her grandmother's house. The songwriter pleads for Olivia to save herself. He specifically asks her not to let her trafficker drag her to an early death, to break the chains of enslavement, and to stop using her body. This song bears a powerful message, however, not for Olivia but rather for us. Olivia cannot save herself without us. Awareness is a must. Victim blaming has to cease as no one chooses to be trafficked. If we are not careful, we can also become hypnotized into thinking trafficking is a legitimate business where the product, girls and women, have the opportunity to choose.

REFERENCES

Anthony, M. (1978). *Olivia, lost and turned out*. Retrieved from http://www.metrolyrics.com/olivia-lost-and-turned-out-lyrics-the-whispers.html; http://www.discogs.com/artist/1024187-Malcolm-Anthony

Banks, D., Kyckelhahn, T., & BJS Statisticians. (2011). *Special Report: Characteristics of suspected human trafficking incidents, 2008–2010*. U.S. Department of Justice, Office of Justice Programs, Bureau of Justice Statistics. Retrieved from http://www.bjs.gov/content/pub/pdf/cshti0810.pdf

Batchelor, V., & Lane, I. (2013). Breaking the code: Domestic minor sex trafficking and school children. In J. Hall (Ed.), *Children's human rights and public schooling in the United States* (pp. 103–115). Rotterdam: Sense Publishers.

Batchelor, V., & Lane, I. (2015). Sex trafficking and black girls: Breaking the code of silence in schools and in our community. In C. F. Collins (Ed.), *Black girls and adolescents: Facing life's challenges* (pp. 220–237). Westport, CT: Praeger Publishers.

Biernacki, P., & Waldorf, D. (1981). Sampling: Problems and techniques of chain referral sampling. *Sociological Methods and Research, 10*(2), 141–163.

Chuang, J. (2006). Beyond a snapshot: Preventing human trafficking in the global economy. *Indiana Journal of Global Legal Studies, 13*(1), Article 5. Retrieved from http://www.repository.law.indiana.edu/ijgls/vol13/iss1/5

Dank, M., Khan, B., Downey, P. M., Kotonias, C., Mayer, D., Owens, C., . . . Yu, L. (2014). Estimating the size and structure of the underground commercial sex economy in eight major U.S. cities. *The Urban Institute*. Retrieved from: http://www.urban.org/UploadedPDF/413047-Underground-Commercial-Sex-Economy.pdf

Emery, A., Heffron, L. C., & Moore, D. (2012). *Human trafficking: Black girls are still enslaved*. Central Texas African American family support conference. Retrieved from http://www.ctaafsc.org/ama/orig/2012_Conference/PPT/pdf/Human_Trafficking_Final__2–11–12.pdf

Finklea, K. M., Fernandes-Alcantara, A. L., & Siskin, A. (2011, June, 21). *Sex trafficking of children in the United States: Overview and issues for Congress*. Congressional Research Service. Retrieved from http://www.fas.org/sgp/crs/misc/R41878.pdf

Girl for Sale. (2010–2013). *Girl for sale & others*. Retrieved from http://www.girlforsale.org/

Gordon, E. (2006). *Black children missing in alarming numbers, for NPR Copyright ©2006*. Retrieved from http://www.npr.org/templates/story/story.php?storyId=5393141

Green, S. J. (2009). Pimp tells of 'selling' girls with dream. *The Seattle Times: Local News*. Retrieved from http://seattletimes.com/html/localnews/2010113369prostitutiontriall22m.html

Jane Doe Inc. (JDI). (2014). *The Massachusetts coalition against sexual assault and domestic violence*. Retrieved from http://www.janedoe.org/learn-more/what-is-vaw

Klein, C. (2013). *The birth of "Stockholm Syndrome," 40 years ago: History in the headlines*. Retrieved from http://www.history.com/news/stockholm-syndrome

Kotrla, K. (2010). Domestic minor sex trafficking in the United States. *Social Work, 55*(2), 181–187.

Mears, A. (2012). Age limits underscore our obsession with youth. *The New York Times: The opinion pages- Room for debate*. Retrieved from http://www.nytimes.com/roomfordebate/2012/09/13/sweet-16-and-a-runway-model/age-limits-for-fashion-models-underscore-our-obsession-with-youth

MSNBC in association with Santoki Productions. (2008). Sex Slaves in the suburbs. New York: NBC Universal Media.

National Conference of State Legislators (NCSL). 2011. *Human trafficking laws in the United States*. Retrieved from http://www.ncsl.org/research/civil-and-criminal-justice/human-trafficking-laws-in-the-states-updated-nov.aspx

Netter, S. *Dad: Shaniya's mom trafficked her to settle drug debt*. Retrieved from http://abcnews.go.com/WN/accused-shaniya-davis-kidnapper-charged-murder-rape/story?id=9136407

Nexstar Broadcasting. (2013). *Study shows sex trafficking has become more profitable than selling drugs*. Retrieved from http://www.localmemphis.com/news/local/story/Study-Shows-Sex-Trafficking-Has-BecomeMore/d/story/t2khCwnCd0S35XFCMoxAHw

Polaris Project. (2010). *Human trafficking statistics*. National Human Trafficking Resource Center. Retrieved from http://www.handsacrosstheworldmn.org/resources/Human+Trafficking+Statistics.pdf

Polaris Project. (2013). *2013 State ratings on human trafficking laws*. Retrieved from http://www.polarisproject.org/what-we-do/policy-advocacy/national-policy/state-ratings-on-human-trafficking-laws

Polaris Project. (2014). *Polaris project: For a world without slavery. Residential brothels*. Retrieved from http://www.polarisproject.org/human-trafficking/sex-trafficking-in-the-us/residential-brothels

Reichert, J., & Sylwestrzak, A. (2013). *National survey of residential programs for victims of sex trafficking.* Retrieved from http://www.icjia.state.il.us/public/pdf/ResearchReports/NSRHVST_101813.pdf

Rescue and Restore Coalition of Louisiana. (2009). *FAQs: Human trafficking stats.* Retrieved from http://www.traffickinghope.org/faqsstats.php

Saar, M. S. (2009). *Shaniya's shame.* Retrieved from http://www.theroot.com/views/shaniyas-shame

SafeNetwork. (2008). *Minnesota center against violence and abuse: Herstory of domestic violence: A timeline of the battered women's movement.* Retrieved from https://people.uvawise.edu/pww8y/Supplement/ConceptsSup/Gender/HerstoryDomV.html#martin

Shared Hope International. (2009). *The national report on domestic minor sex trafficking: America's prostituted children.* Retrieved from http://sharedhope.org/wpcontent/uploads/2012/09/SHI_National_Report_on_DMST_2009without_cover.pdf FORMATTING ISSUE

Three 6 Mafia. (2005). *"It's hard out here for a pimp" in Hustle & Flow.* Retrieved from http://slangcity.com/songs/its_hard_out_here_for_a_pimp.htm

Tillet, S. (2010). *Black girls are still enslaved: The sexual trafficking of our young females is happening at an alarming rate. Who will free them?* Retrieved from http://www.theroot.com/views/black-girls-are-still-enslaved

United Nations. (2000). *Protocol to prevent, suppress and punish trafficking in persons, especially women and children, supplementing the United Nations convention against transnational organized crime* (General Assembly resolution 55/25). New York: United Nations General Assembly.

United Nations Children's Fund (UNICEF). (2000, May). Domestic violence against women and girls. *Innocent Digest* .6. Retrieved from http:www.hawaii.edu/hivandaids/Domestic%20Violence%20Against%20Women%20and%20Girls.pdf

United Nations Office on Drugs and Crime (2004). United Nations Convention against transnational organized crime and the protocols thereto. United Nations, New York http://www.unodc.org/documents/middleeastandnorthafrica/organised-crime/UNITED_NATIONS_CONVENTION_AGAINST_TRANSNATIONAL_ORGANIZED_CRIME_AND_THE_PROTOCOLS_THERETO.pdf

U.S. Department of State. (2013). *The State Department 2013 trafficking in persons report.* Retrieved from http://www.state.gov/j/tip/rls/rm/2013/211833.htm

Williamson, C., Perdue, T., Belton, L., Burns, O., Barrows, J., Smouse, T., . . . Michel, E. (2012). *Domestic sex trafficking in Ohio: Research & analysis sub-committee.* Ohio Human Trafficking Commission. Retrieved from http://www.ohioattorneygeneral.gov/getattachment/2ff15706-77ad-4567-b1aa-d8330b5c4005/2012-Domestic-Sex-Trafficking-in-Ohio-Report.aspx

3 Longitudinal Ethnography: Uncovering Domestic Abuse in Low-Income Women's Lives

Linda M. Burton, Diane Purvin, and Raymond Garrett-Peters

Many family science and human development scholars argue that it is critically important to examine women's histories of physical and sexual abuse in studies of their life course. Yet, given the sensitivity of this topic and respondents' tendency to withhold troubling information about themselves, it is difficult to gather accurate and detailed information about the prevalence and nature of these experiences in women's lives (see Jouriles, McDonald, Norwood, & Ezell, 2001). For example, panel surveys of life course and family transitions, such as the National Survey of Families and Households and the Panel Study of Income Dynamics, either do not include questions about abuse or they employ less than ideal measures that result in significant underreporting of these experiences. Moreover, studies such as the National Violence Against Women surveys are designed specifically to identify the prevalence of abuse, but they do not gather information about processes (e.g., nuanced behaviors and styles of communication) involved in women's disclosures of abuse (Bachman & Saltzman, 1995; Finkelhor, 1994). Overall, most surveys rely on limited measures that fail to capture the full range of women's subjective experiences of abuse, or they neglect to consider abuse as a phenomenon affecting the entire life course of women and their families (Macmillan, 2001; Williams, 2003). Such problems in measurement and assessment impede our understanding of abuse prevalence and the ways it shapes the life course of women, particularly low-income women who face heightened vulnerabilities from its effects (Leone, Johnson, Cohan, & Lloyd, 2004; Sokoloff & Dupont, 2005).

Compared to surveys, ethnographic studies often find themselves "knee-deep" in data about women's physical and sexual abuse experiences. In many ethnographies, such issues typically emerge naturalistically as unanticipated themes during data collection. For instance, in ethnographic studies seeking to understand the life course of low-income women, researchers reported that although they did not specifically solicit information about abuse, it was a disturbingly common experience for their respondents, a fact of family life to be negotiated, along with the other, numerous challenges of poverty (Butler & Burton, 1990; Dodson, 1998; Fine & Weis, 1998; Musick, 1993). And, more recently, large-scale studies of welfare reform that include ethnographic components have reported the emergence of abuse issues as unanticipated yet significant factors influencing outcomes of interest (Cherlin, Burton, Hurt, & Purvin 2004; Scott, London, & Myers, 2002). These studies suggest that abuse, a highly influential force in low-income mothers' lives, is likely to go undetected in studies that neither address it directly nor employ sensitive enough methods to capture it naturalistically. In light of these findings, we ask the following questions: Could ethnography be one of the most useful and important methods for gathering accurate data about the prevalence of physical and sexual abuse in the life course of low-income women? What processes are involved when women reveal histories of physical and sexual abuse through ethnography?

In this chapter, we address these questions using longitudinal ethnographic data from *Welfare, Children, and Families: A Three-City Study* (hereafter, the Three-City Study). In this ethnography (described in greater detail later in this chapter) we sought to understand the life course experiences of 256 African American, Hispanic, and non-Hispanic white low-income mothers of young children in Boston, Chicago, and San Antonio over a 6-year period following the implementation of welfare reform. We begin this discussion with a brief overview of the features of ethnography that render it a viable life course method for gathering accurate and detailed data about physical and sexual abuse in women's lives. We then describe the processes involved in uncovering women's abuse experiences in the Three-City Study ethnography. In doing so, we illustrate the degree to which experiences of physical and sexual abuse permeate the lives of low-income mothers, and present methodological and ethical challenges to ethnographers. Our process of uncovering abuse in women's lives was characterized by distinctive respondent disclosure patterns evoked by certain trigger topics, recent crisis events in respondents' lives, and ethnographers' direct inquiries. The disclosure experiences also involved ethnographers' own emotional reactions and ethical responsibilities toward the respondents. The implications of these disclosure processes for research designs and methodological issues concerning life course research on low-income women also are discussed.

ETHNOGRAPHY AND REVEALING EXPERIENCES OF PHYSICAL AND SEXUAL ABUSE

Very few people are completely revealing in what they do and say in the presence of others. This claim applies to passing interactants on a city sidewalk; close, lifelong friends; or even respondents answering a sociological survey. As social learning theorists would argue, all individuals are socialized to be mindful of some normative set of rules regarding thoughts, feelings, and behaviors gleaned through their participation in social life. Goffman (1959, 1963), with his emphasis on phenomena such as impression management, stigma, and passing, to name but a few, sheds important light on this universal human tendency to guard the information we reveal to others. A main reason for this lack of disclosure is that people learn, both explicitly and implicitly, that their communication of information about self, others, thoughts, and actions can have consequences, both negative and positive (Blumer, 1955; Deutscher, 1966; Schwalbe, 1987). With this in mind, people often try to craft desired images of self, limit the kind and amount of information they share, and hide sensitive or discrediting information from others. And so, alcoholics may attempt to hide signs of inappropriate drinking; workers sometimes cover up evidence of laziness or mistakes to bosses; family members may reveal limited information about one another to outsiders; and women may hide or minimize experiences of sexual and physical abuse.

As social scientists intent on learning as much as possible from those we study, how are we to deal with this potential problem? And, more specifically, how can we gain access to important information, such as women's histories of being physically or sexually abused, especially when that data can better inform the understanding and interpretation of their life course circumstances? We argue that ethnographic research is an especially valuable means for gaining access to these types of sensitive data. The depth of information that emanates from longitudinal ethnography moves us closer than most data-collection methods to uncovering sensitive and hidden experiences that shape individuals' life course (Smith, Tessaro, & Earp, 1995). Ethnography allows for the discovery of such experiences in at least two ways. First, it enables researchers to collect a wide range of data by actually being there, over time, with those being studied to observe and question individuals under the conditions in which they usually act. Second, ethnographic research enables fieldworkers, through the development of trust and rapport with those studied, to elicit data on sensitive information in participants' lives—information that is less likely to be revealed in any single or limited number of encounters.

"BEING THERE"

Ethnographic research, and fieldwork in particular, is a necessarily social research practice (see Gans, 1968; Gold, 1958; Jarvie, 1969; Stebbins, 1972; Vidich, 1955). Unlike other methods of social research, ethnographic fieldwork entails actually inserting oneself, to varying degrees, into the lives of the people being studied (see Clarke, 1975). In the course of doing research, ethnographers are inevitably enmeshed in social relationships with those studied by virtue of participating in the latter's activities. Asher and Fine (1991, p. 196), in their study of women married to alcoholics, underscore this feature of ethnographic research:

> Good field research inevitably involves the creation and cultivation of relationships. These relationships will, depending upon the goals of the

research and the types of persons whom one is studying, take many forms, but in all cases there must be both a measure of personal caring and respect and an interpersonal distance that derives from the separate roles and social worlds of researcher and informant.

Any given ethnographic research project likewise comprises a series of social acts and relations, a history of cumulative acts that also entails the roles, identities, interactional pressures, and normative social obligations attendant to any set of social relationships (see Emerson & Pollner, 2001; Singer, Hertas, & Scott, 2000). Here, ethnography also stands out as social practice, precisely because of the need to cultivate and maintain relationships with those being studied, often over long periods of time (see Cassell & Wax, 1980; Clarke, 1975; Harrington, 2003).

As typically practiced, ethnographic study involves the close-up and detailed reporting of what people do and say in the flow of everyday activities. It is achieved through some mix of observation, participant observation, and formal and informal interviewing (see Agar, 1996; Spradley, 1980). Likewise, ethnographic research functions as a kind of ongoing, joint accomplishment with those individuals or groups studied, one in which fieldworkers are compelled to manage relationships, identities, and emotions as they attempt to maintain their good standing relative to the individuals and groups they are studying (see Kleinman, 1991; Kleinman & Copp, 1993). As a result, much of the epistemic and analytic power of ethnographic research comes from "having been there," from observing individuals or groups of people acting under conditions in which they usually act, and from describing a social world from the perspective of those who inhabit it (see Becker, 1996; Duneier, 2007).

It is in this sense of being there, and being there over extended periods of time, that ethnographic research serves as a useful way of getting at sensitive or potentially hidden behaviors. Part of this advantage derives from doing sustained ethnographic fieldwork that provides opportunities for collecting data as people go through their daily rounds across different settings and activities. Another particularly epistemological advantage comes from fieldworkers' actual participation in activities with research participants. Such participation (i.e., participant observation) provides opportunities to engage in close observation and questioning of social actors as they go about their lives, adapt to their particular circumstances, and provide understandings from the perspectives of those inhabiting distinct social worlds—worlds that typically are distinct from those of academic researchers (see, e.g., Burton 1990, 1997; Burton, Obeidallah, & Allison, 1996).

Rather than relying solely on what people tell them, for instance, in formal interviews, ethnographic fieldworkers are able to supplement, and, hence, to provide a check against these data in the course of doing participant observation and informal questioning. Thus, occasions can arise in which ethnographers experience contradictions between what people tell them and what they actually observe people doing or hear reported from others. The reasons for these contradictions, as discussed earlier, can be many: a desire to hide potentially embarrassing information; a fuzzy memory during formal interviewing; or even the phraseology of a particular interview question by an ethnographer. Regardless of the bases, by being there over time and participating in the social world being studied, fieldworkers gain opportunities to uncover new, contradictory, and potentially illuminating forms of data (see also Duneier, 2007).

BUILDING TRUST AND RAPPORT

Ethnographic fieldwork also enables researchers to get at sensitive and hidden data in another way: by being there when research participants are ready to reveal previously concealed information on their own terms. Because many forms of sensitive data, such as experiences of physical and sexual abuse, are kept hidden by research participants, such data can be difficult to obtain, at least until researchers have earned some measure of trust (Dodson & Schmalzbauer, 2005; Wax, 1956). Sincere promises of confidentiality and anonymity can go some distance toward convincing participants to share sensitive data, but these measures are sometimes not enough. In settings in which those studied are concerned about revealing too much of themselves, not until a long-term, comfortable relationship has been established do research participants share information with ethnographers that could potentially have others see them in a less favorable light.

Part of this strength of ethnographic research to elicit sensitive data is a product of participants' felt obligations to reciprocate toward ethnographers in what has become over time a sustained relationship. Part of it derives from fieldworkers' willingness to serve as sympathetic listeners in the course of these cumulative interactions. Either way, central to such sustained relationships are feelings of trust and rapport that fieldworkers are able to establish and maintain with those they are studying. When trust and rapport are established, research participants often reveal sensitive information in the course of "altercasting" (Goffman, 1959; Weinstein & Deutschberger, 1963) fieldworkers into the role of therapeutic listener, someone to whom they can voice their fears and problems in confidence (see, e.g., Ortiz, 2004; Wax, 1956). This ability is made possible given an ethnographer's facility to listen without judgment and to make and keep promises of confidentiality—that is, to instill a sense of trust in the research participant. And for an ethnographer who comes to the research setting as an outsider, lack of involvement in the participant's immediate social world can make him or her all the more attractive (Kloos, 1969; Pollner & Emerson, 1983). In this context, ethnographers come to represent a special category of acquaintance or friend who, not bound up in the participant's network of close relationships, is not likely to spread gossip and create trouble.

DESCRIPTION OF THE THREE-CITY STUDY

To illustrate the processes involved in how ethnography can facilitate uncovering physical and sexual abuse in the lives of low-income women we draw on data from the Three-City Study, a longitudinal, multisite, multimethod project designed to examine the impact of welfare reform on the lives of low-income African American, Latino, Hispanic, and non-Hispanic white families and their young children (for a detailed description of the research design of the ethnography, see Winston et al., 1999). Study participants resided in poor neighborhoods in Boston, Chicago, and San Antonio. In addition to longitudinal surveys of a random sample comprising 2,402 families, and an embedded developmental study of 700 families, the Three-City Study included an ethnography of 256 families and their children. These families were not in the survey sample but resided in the same neighborhoods as survey respondents.

SAMPLE DESCRIPTION

Families were recruited into the ethnography between June 1999 and December 2000. Recruitment sites include formal child care settings (e.g., Head Start), the WIC (Women, Infants and Children) program, neighborhood community centers, local welfare offices, churches, and other public assistance agencies. Of the 256 families who participated in the ethnography, 212 families were selected if they included a child age 2–4 to ensure sample comparability with the survey and embedded developmental samples. To inform our understanding of how welfare reform was affecting families with disabilities, the other 44 ethnographic families were recruited specifically because they had a child age 0–8 years with a moderate or severe disability. At the time of enrollment in the ethnography, all families had household incomes at or below 200% of the federal poverty line (U.S. Department of Health and Human Services, 1999).

Table 3.1 describes demographic characteristics of the mothers in the ethnographic sample. The majority of mothers (42%) were of Latino or Hispanic

Table 3.1   Sample Characteristics: Three-City Study Ethnography Sample

Characteristic	N	%[a]
City		
Boston	71	28
Chicago	95	37
San Antonio	90	35
Ethnicity/race		
African American	98	38

Characteristic	N	%[a]
Latino/Hispanic	108	42
Non-Hispanic white	50	20
Ages of primary caregivers		
15–19	21	8
20–24	67	26
25–29	62	24
30–34	36	14
35–39	35	14
40+	35	14
Education		
Less than high school	110	43
Completed high school or GED	67	26
College or trade school	79	31
TANF/work status		
TANF/working	40	16
TANF/not working	85	33
Non-TANF/working	64	25
Non-TANF/not working	67	26
Number of children primary caregiver is responsible for		
1 child	64	25
2 children	70	27
3 children	63	25
> 4 children	59	23
Children's ages		
< 2	190	28
2–4	174	25
5–9	205	30
10–14	88	13
15–18	28	4
Total	685	
Marital status/living arrangements[b]		
Not married, not cohabiting	142	56
Married, spouse in home	42	17
Married, spouse not in home/separated	24	10
Cohabiting (any marital status)	43	17

Note. N = 256.
[a] Percentages may not sum to 100 due to rounding.
[b] There are missing data for five cases in this category.

ethnicity, with the largest groups being Mexican American, Puerto Rican, and Dominican, in that order. Over half of the mothers were age 29 or younger when they enrolled in the study and a majority had a high school diploma (GED), or had attended a trade school or college. Forty-nine percent of the mothers were receiving welfare (Temporary Assistance for Needy Families [TANF]) when they entered the study; one-third of these were also working. The 256 mothers identified a total of 685 children in their households, with most children under 4 years of age. Most mothers indicated that they were neither married nor cohabiting at the start of the study. However, longitudinal interviews and observations of the sample over time revealed that more respondents were in marital or cohabiting relationships than they had initially reported.

ETHNOGRAPHIC METHODOLOGY

To gather and to analyze ethnographic data on the mothers and their families, a method of "structured discovery" was devised to systematize and to coordinate the efforts of the Three-City Study ethnography team (Burton, Skinner, & Matthews, 2005; Winston et al., 1999). An integrated and transparent process was developed for collecting, handling, and analyzing data that involved consistent input from over 215 ethnographers, qualitative data analysts, and research scientists who worked on the project over the course of 6 years. Interviews with and observations of the respondents focused on specific topics but allowed flexibility to capture unexpected findings and relationships among variables. The interviews covered a wide variety of topics, including intimate relationships; health and health care access; family economics; support networks; and neighborhood environments. Ethnographers also engaged in participant observation with respondents, which included attending family functions and outings; being party to extended conversations and witnessing relationship milestones (e.g., a couple's decision to cohabit) between mothers and their partners; and accompanying mothers and their children to the welfare office, hospital, day care, or workplace, noting both context and interactions in each situation. In 92% of the cases, ethnographers were racially matched with respondents and remained the families' ethnographers for the duration of the study. In most cases, interviews and participant observations were conducted in English, with the exception of 34 families who preferred Spanish. Ethnographers met with each family once or twice per month for 12–18 months, then every 6 months thereafter through 2003. Respondents were compensated with grocery or department store vouchers for each interview or participant observation.

DATA SOURCES

The ethnography generated multiple sources of data that we used to identify processes in uncovering patterns of physical and sexual abuse within the sample. Ethnographers in each city wrote detailed fieldnotes about their interviews and participant observations with families, and all interviews were tape-recorded and transcribed. In addition, we consulted transcripts of principal investigators' group and individual discussions with ethnographers and qualitative data analysts about the families in this analysis. [During the data-collection process, we held monthly cross-site Thought-Provoking Questions (TPQ) conference calls with ethnographers and qualitative data analysts. The purpose of these conference calls was discussion of emergent themes in ethnographers' ongoing field observations and data analysts' synthesis of ethnographers' fieldnotes and transcribed interviews.] All sources of data were coded collaboratively [according to a general thematic coding scheme developed by the principal investigators] by ethnographers and qualitative data analysts for entry into a qualitative data management (QDM) software application, then summarized into detailed case profiles of each family. The QDM program and case profiles enabled counts across the entire sample, as well as detailed analyses of individual cases. When we use specific case examples in this chapter, the mothers and their family members have been assigned pseudonyms.

UNCOVERING PHYSICAL AND SEXUAL ABUSE: THE THREE-CITY STUDY ETHNOGRAPHIC PROCESS

Although our ethnographic methods generated information on a variety of topics related to women's life course experiences, it is important to note that this ethnographic study was not explicitly designed to examine issues of domestic violence or sexual abuse in women's lives. Women's reports of abuse emerged naturalistically in the course of interactions with the ethnographers. When stories of abuse experiences began to surface early in the data-collection process in all three cities, the research team initiated a series of discussions about how to address these disclosures and observations. Principal investigators, senior ethnographers, data analysts, and family ethnographers met online and in conference calls to address a variety of ethical, empirical, and methodological dilemmas posed by "uncovering these experiences," and to develop procedures to protect the physical and emotional safety of both respondents and ethnographers.

During these discussions, those most directly involved in data collection (family ethnographers) emphasized the great degree to which they observed domestic violence and sexual abuse affecting respondent families. Informed by their concerns, the senior project staff requested that data collectors and analysts pay special attention to these issues, and attempt to document and understand their impact on women's and their families' lives, and their relationship to specific outcomes. As a result, the Three-City Study ethnography generated considerable interview and observational data on the patterns and effects of domestic violence and sexual abuse among low-income families over time and across generations. In efforts to analyze and disseminate these data, researchers affiliated with the study sought to place these findings in the context of prior research. Literature reviews conducted for this chapter, as well as for recently published articles (Cherlin et al., 2004; Purvin, 2003, 2007) and an article in press (Burton, Cherlin, Winn, Estacion, & Holder-Taylor, in press), indicate that issues of domestic violence and sexual abuse have not been adequately addressed in general studies of the lives of low-income women, and that gathering data on, measuring, and appropriately interpreting the incidence and processes of physical and sexual abuse among low-income women is complicated and difficult in practice.

THE PREVALENCE OF ABUSE

Over the course of the study we determined that the prevalence of physical and sexual abuse experiences in mothers' lives was considerably higher than we had ever anticipated. Sexual abuse included mothers' reports of rape, molestation, parentally enforced child prostitution, and witnessing incest acts. Physical abuse comprised physical beatings, attacks with weapons, and witnessing consistent physical violence among parents, partners, and children. Drawing on existing studies that underscore the impact of witnessing sexual abuse and domestic violence on the life course (Feerick & Haugaard, 1999; Luster, Small, & Lower, 2002; Straus, 1992), and the severity of the exposure in our sample, we purposely included "witnessing experiences" in the sexual and physical abuse categories. Mothers' reports of witnessing sexual abuse or domestic violence of short duration or questionable intensity (e.g., "I saw my mother's boyfriend slap her one time") were not included in the analysis. However, witnessing experiences, such as the one recounted by Noel, a 34-year-old mother of five, were included:

"My sister and I slept in the same bedroom in bunk beds. I slept on the top bunk and my sister on the bottom. Every night for as long as I can remember, my father would come to my sister's bed and force her to have sex with him. I lay there and listened quietly."

With respect to the incidence of physical violence, in most cases the violence was directed toward women and children by men, but in three instances women were perpetrators as well. For example, Serena, a 35-year-old mother, suspected her abusive partner of cheating on her and "followed him to the club with a gun." They argued, she pulled the gun on him, and in the struggle that ensued, Serena's partner was shot in the hand. Serena was charged with assault with a deadly weapon and received 2 years' probation.

Most mothers who reported sexual abuse also reported physical abuse, suggesting that sexual abuse often occurred in the context of physical violence. As Table 3.2 indicates, 36% of the mothers disclosed that they had been sexually and physically abused; 3% revealed that they had only been sexually abused (primarily in childhood), and 26% said they had only been physically abused (primarily in domestic violence situations as adults). In 35% of the cases, mothers reported that they had not been sexually or

Table 3.2 Percent Distribution of Physical and Sexual Abuse: Three-City Study Ethnography

History of physical and sexual abuse	% distribution[a]
None	35
Sexual abuse	3
Physical abuse	26
Sexual and physical abuse	36
Total %	100

Note. N = 228. Total ethnography sample N = 256 (28 cases were not included in this analysis because of insufficient data).
[a] Percentages do not sum to 100 due to rounding.

physically abused in their lifetimes. It is possible, of course, that some of these mothers may also have experienced abuse but were reluctant to mention it. Still, the extended duration of the fieldwork and the trust that developed between the ethnographers and respondents make it likely that our reports are more complete than many other studies.

PATTERNS OF DISCLOSING PHYSICAL AND SEXUAL ABUSE

Overall, 64% (N = 147) of the mothers who participated in the ethnography disclosed that they had been sexually abused or had experienced physical abuse in childhood, adulthood, or both. What we found intriguing, and what we hope scholars who study life courses of women will find useful, are the ways in which the ethnographers uncovered mothers' histories of abuse.

Data on sexual abuse and domestic violence were gathered from mothers through a number of emergent approaches. For example, after several mothers revealed abuse experiences in early interviews with ethnographers, we developed specific questions in the interview protocol concerning lifetime sexual abuse and domestic violence experiences. Some mothers revealed their experiences to ethnographers in response to these questions, but most did so in response to questions about related topics (e.g., intimate relationships), others in the context of unrelated topics (e.g., discussions about housing), and still others as a function of experiencing recent episodes of abuse.

Three patterns of participant disclosure of abuse were apparent in the ethnographic data: trigger topics disclosure, crisis or recent event disclosure, and ethnographer-prompted disclosure. Of the mothers who disclosed a history of physical and/or sexual abuse to the ethnographers, 71% demonstrated the trigger topics disclosure pattern; 19%, the crisis or recent event pattern; and 10%, ethnographer-prompted disclosure.

TRIGGER TOPICS DISCLOSURE

The "trigger topics disclosure" pattern involved mothers unexpectedly revealing their sexual abuse and domestic violence histories to ethnographers when they were asked about not only related topics, such as health and intimate relationships, but also seemingly unrelated topics, such as transportation, family demographics, and intergenerational caregiving. For instance, general questions about health, particularly stress and coping, often triggered mothers' disclosures of sexual abuse and domestic violence experiences. The conversation between Sonya, a 37-year-old African American mother of three, and her ethnographer during a health interview is illustrative:

> ETHNOGRAPHER: What would you say was the biggest source of stress for you in the past year?
>
> SONYA: Dealing with a man [referring to her son's father, William]. They can really put you in a depressed stage. Here I am doing what I know is right with my kids, then this one person goin' try to come in and try to tell you another way, which, he just want to be the head of the household and treat you like you just nobody. And I couldn't go for that. . . . It was eating me up inside.
>
> ETHNOGRAPHER: OK. . . . Let's talk more about William.
>
> SONYA: He's crazy. . . . He was really jealous and just crazy. I had headaches daily when he was in the house. I was depressed, but I didn't take medication or nothing. My sister had told me to get rid of him. I was brainwashed though. He told me not to see my family because they didn't like him. I fell for it. He had me so stressed out. My pregnancy with Dante was hard, because I was sick.
>
> ETHNOGRAPHER: You were sick?
>
> SONYA: Yeah, he had been sleeping around and gave me gonorrhea. I'm still embarrassed talking about it. Sometimes I didn't want to sleep with him, but he'd rape me. I told him I was gonna' call the police and he said, "Go ahead. Ain't nobody gonna' arrest me for wanting to be with my woman."

In subsequent interviews, Sonya described in great detail the physical violence and sexual abuse she had experienced from other partners, as well as those experienced by her young daughter.

During Darlene's health interview, which was conducted by the ethnographer during her seventh monthly visit to Darlene's home, the ethnographer asked Darlene how she coped with stress. This 26-year-old Latina mother of four responded:

"I used to keep a journal of my life, because, when I was younger, I was molested. And so was my sister, so you know, one of our things of therapy was, you know, to write down what we felt for the next time we [would see] our counselor, and I was just like, all right, you know, well, and then I just kept a habit of constantly writing. . . ."

Darlene, like Sonya, went on, in several interviews thereafter, to provide explicit descriptions of her abuse experiences.

Liza, a 28-year-old mother of three, initially revealed her experiences with abuse when the ethnographer accompanied her to a doctor's appointment. At this appointment, Liza learned that her last Pap smear was abnormal. When asked about her sexual history, Liza noted that she was primarily intimate with her husband. The ethnographer seized the opportunity to ask her how she met her husband. Liza stated that this was a funny story. She nonchalantly recounted that she met her husband after having just ended a relationship with a man who broke her nose. This information was disclosed on the ethnographer's seventh visit with Liza.

Interview topics, such as work, transportation, residential mobility, and household composition, also triggered abuse disclosures from some respondents. For example, during the 23rd visit to the home of Delilah, a 40-year-old European American divorcée and mother of four children, the ethnographer conducted a follow-up interview concerning Delilah's past and current work experiences. Although she had failed to mention particulars about her work history in previous interviews, after 2 years of interviews, Delilah finally told the ethnographer that in the past she had worked at a bank as a switchboard operator until her former husband physically injured her. Delilah stated: "I went to work with a black eye. People at the bank noticed. When it happened a second time, I felt embarrassed coming to work, so I quit like cold turkey. And I really didn't like that idea 'cause, you know, it leaves you in a status of not good standing."

Residential history interviews also prompted disclosures of abuse. The following conversation between Estella, a 30-year-old Latina mother of three, and her ethnographer took place during a residential history interview. Estella had in fact mentioned to the ethnographer in a previous interview that as a child she had witnessed her mother being abused. The discussion of her former residences, however, prompted further disclosure:

ETHNOGRAPHER: So you remember that home, in that area.
ESTELLA: Umm, in that area.
ETHNOGRAPHER: You were like 7, 8 years old then?

ESTELLA: And, then I remember another one in [another city], right off of [street]. It was beautiful, too; it was called [name of development]. And I used to live there; we used to live out there. And, let's see how many more places I can remember.

ETHNOGRAPHER: But you don't have any one place in particular that would bring you memories.

ESTELLA: Yeah, there's one that's a sad memory, because I remember my mother being abused, between two men. One was her ex-husband and another was her boyfriend . . . and another one where me and my sister were molested by my mother's ex-boyfriend. So it's like there's places that, you know, I remember that are bad, and then there's some places.

ETHNOGRAPHER: Different places or the same place?

ESTELLA: Right, different places, and I just remember places where they were happy places, where I can remember.

Gathering demographic information on marital histories also triggered abuse disclosures from mothers. Marital history interviews were generally conducted during the second monthly visit. Thus, when Marilyn, a 45-year-old European American mother of four, discussed her abuse experiences during a marital history interview, she became one of the study's earliest disclosers of abuse:

"So for 6 years I was married to him, well, not married to him. We got married for a year, and it didn't work out. We always fought, and then we renewed our vows for another year and that didn't work out. Sometime before she [Marilyn's daughter] was born he was very abusive. . . . [There is an extended silence before Marilyn continued on with her story.] He beat me up when I was pregnant with her. So I've been divorced since after she was born. . . . He physically and mentally abused me. He locked me in my apartment, in my bedroom. He told me if he wanted to, he could rape me. He said, 'Might as well get charged with something.' He gave me a couple of hits in the face, hit my head on the headboard, which was glass. I ended up with a contusion and went to the hospital for premature labor."

On the next visit to the home, the ethnographer learned that Marilyn's two youngest children had been sexually abused by her current boyfriend. In the 3 weeks that ensued, the police removed Les, Marilyn's cohabiting boyfriend, from the home for committing these crimes. Despite these very sensitive disclosures and unfolding events, Marilyn remained in the study for 6 years, until its completion.

CRISIS DISCLOSURE

The crisis or recent event disclosure pattern occurred when the ethnographer unexpectedly "walked in" on a domestic violence situation when visiting the participant, or when the participant experienced a sexual abuse or domestic violence episode a few days or weeks prior to the ethnographer's regularly scheduled visit. In both instances, the abuse situation was "fresh" in the minds of mothers, and they chose to discuss it with their ethnographers in great detail. In most of these cases, the ethnographers suspected abuse (as indicated in ethnographers' fieldnotes and in discussions with their supervisors and team members), but they did not feel that they could ask the participant about it directly until the crisis-prompted disclosure. For example, Janine, the ethnographer for Patrice, a 28-year-old European mother of two, describes the circumstances that led to Patrice's crisis-prompted disclosure:

> "I arrived at Patrice's house 10 minutes before the interview only to find the streets covered with cops, patrol cars, and an ambulance.
> 'Oh my God,' I thought. 'What has happened?' They were taking one man out of Patrice's house. He appeared to be shot or stabbed. Patrice was on the porch screaming, her face bloody and cut. The kids were running around everywhere screaming and crying. . . . I feared that my worst suspicions about the prevalence of domestic violence in Patrice's life were about to be confirmed. . . . When I visited Patrice 3 weeks later the floodgate opened without me asking. I listened as she told me everything about the incident, and about other incidents of physical and sexual abuse she had experienced nonstop since childhood."

ETHNOGRAPHER-PROMPTED DISCLOSURE

The third pattern, ethnographer-prompted disclosure, reflects situations in which ethnographers directly asked mothers about their past and current experiences with sexual abuse or domestic violence. Ethnographers usually asked direct questions about these topics in an interview if they noticed a behavioral reaction from mothers when discussing their intimate relationships with their partners. One ethnographer's interview with Samantha, a 28-year-old European American mother of two, is illustrative:

> "When Samantha was telling me how she met Charles [her current husband], she said that her breakup from her daughter's father Byron was 'a whole big mess.' The expression on her face and the way she said it sent up a red flag for me, so I wanted to ask her more about it. I asked her whether, when she had split up with Byron, there was anything dangerous about it, or whether it was just upsetting in general. Samantha said, 'He was very violent, um, and then I found out he was cheatin' on me with a younger girl; at the time I was what, 20, 21, and he was

about 23 goin' out with a 15-year-old, so . . . I just had it. He was very abusive, and I couldn't take it anymore anyways, so that just made me get the strength to say, 'Get out of my house.' "

The ethnographer asked whether Byron was abusive the whole time Samantha was with him. Samantha replied:

"No, um, actually it didn't start until, um, the beginnin' of when I was pregnant. He didn't know I was pregnant; I didn't neither at the time, and then it stopped for awhile, and then after I had my daughter, it started up bad. 'Cause I didn't think, he didn't wanna be a family guy, you know, the responsibilities, so, and that's it. He hasn't seen my daughter since she was 2."

Samantha got two restraining orders on him after they broke up. After Samantha met Charles, about 7 months after she and Byron broke up, Byron would call up and threaten Samantha, and he would drive by her house. Later in this interview, and again in the intimate relationship interview, Samantha described in explicit detail the numerous bruises and injuries she received from Byron, and the effects of his abuse on her oldest daughter, who was exposed to it as an infant. Although Samantha initially described her current husband as not abusive, in an incident about a year after this, he became violent and she called the cops. I met with her about a week later, and she described to me what had happened in the course of explaining what had changed since our last meeting.

TIMING OF DISCLOSURE

It is important to note that there was a range in the timing of disclosure, with approximately 12% of the mothers who revealed physical and sexual abuse experiences telling their stories to the ethnographers during visits or participant observations in the first 3 months of their involvement in the study. Twenty-nine percent disclosed physical and sexual abuse experiences during the 4 to 6-month visits with the ethnographers, 40% during the 7 to 9-month visits, and 19% after 10 to 24 visits. The variation in disclosure timing reflects a range of "turning points" between the mothers and the ethnographers. A turning point is the precise moment in time when the participant trusts the ethnographer enough to share intimate, highly sensitive, and often painful information, such as a history of sexual abuse.

ETHNOGRAPHERS' REACTIONS AND RESPONSIBILITIES TO PARTICIPANTS

As the Three-City Study ethnographic data illustrate, the elements of ethnography that enable it to uncover experiences of physical and sexual abuse so effectively also present ethical and interpersonal challenges (see Becker-Blease & Freyd, 2006; Dodson & Schmalzbauer, 2005). Ethnographers, as we noted earlier, are very likely to find themselves in privileged positions vis-à-vis their informants by virtue of their roles as empathetic and supportive listeners who become, at least temporarily, trusted personal confidantes, yet are not bound up in participants' social networks. Although effective and ethical researchers prepare for and develop protocols to address such potential issues of blurred interpersonal boundaries and disclosure, physical and sexual abuse create unique dilemmas for researchers engaged in ethnographic data collection, analysis, and interpretation. In the Three-City Study ethnography, two dilemmas are particularly noteworthy: vicarious trauma and safety.

VICARIOUS TRAUMA

Chief among Three-City Study ethnographers' reactions to participants' disclosure of abuse was secondary or vicarious trauma. Developed as a construct based in large part on the experiences of counselors working with victims and survivors of sexual assault and domestic abuse (Schauben & Frazier, 1995), "vicarious trauma" refers to the negative emotional and psychic impact on those "empathically engaged with clients' trauma material" (Pearlman & Saakvitne, 1995, p. 31). Because intensive qualitative interviews can be analogous to therapeutic interactions (Birch & Miller, 2000; Gale, 1992), ethnographers engaged in fieldwork with victims and survivors of traumas such as domestic and sexual abuse, particularly those who have not previously acknowledged or disclosed their experiences, are perhaps as likely as actual counselors to become recipients of such trauma disclosures. The potential for vicarious trauma in intensive qualitative research is just beginning to be addressed in the literature (Etherington, 2007).

Although the majority of sexual assault and domestic violence counselors do not become secondarily traumatized to an incapacitating degree, research suggests that significant numbers experience at least some formal symptoms of vicarious trauma (Bride, 2007; Schauben & Frazier, 1995). There is currently no information on the prevalence of vicarious trauma among researchers working with traumatized persons. However, the levels reported among counselors suggest that vicarious trauma is a potentially significant risk for ethnographers engaged in fieldwork with trauma victims or survivors. Recent work (see Etherington, 2007), as well as our experience on the Three-City Study ethnography, indicates that all research staff who engage intensively with narrative data on the trauma of physical and sexual abuse are potentially vulnerable to vicarious trauma. This includes data transcribers, coders, and analysts who may or may not have conducted direct data collection or fieldwork themselves. Within the Three-City Study team, our data analysts, who did not collect data but were coding it and writing family profiles, frequently had "melt downs," which included "having to pull off on the side of the road on the way home from work to have a good cry," "staying in bed all day because I just couldn't believe someone could do this to another person," or "sitting on the curb with two other ethnographers and just crying my eyes out because I didn't know what else to do."

SAFETY

An additional ethical and potentially methodological dilemma posed by the emergence of physical and sexual abuse in data collection is the problem of safety. Through their privileged positions of confidence, fieldworkers may become aware of threats to the physical safety of both informants and vulnerable others in the community, such as children. Such situations can potentially generate ethical quandaries over whether and how to break confidentiality and disclose threats of violence to outsiders, particularly in the context of mandatory reporting requirements in the event of child abuse or adult domestic violence. Additionally, the safety of fieldworkers themselves may be threatened when they are present in homes where there is the potential for violence, or if they are viewed as allies to persons who are the target of violence or abuse. Such incidents occurred numerous times in the Three-City Study ethnography. For example, one ethnographer observed a drug deal in a respondent's home and was threatened with murder. Another discovered that a respondent was being abused by her husband and was informed by the respondent's mother to "stay away and don't tell anyone what you saw or our family will fix you." Obviously, taking steps to protect the lives and well-being of those at potential risk is paramount, and any questions pertaining to the ethics of breaking confidentiality must be subsumed. Depending on the particular circumstances and the actions taken, the unfolding of such conditions in the course of data collection can create methodological dilemmas with respect to the nature of data collected, the relationship of the fieldworker to the informants and/or the setting, and implications for data analysis and interpretation.

SUMMARY AND CONCLUSION: RESEARCH DESIGN AND METHODOLOGICAL RECOMMENDATIONS IN UNCOVERING ABUSE

Using longitudinal ethnographic data from the Three-City Study, we have described the aspects of ethnography that render it a viable life course methodology for gathering accurate and detailed data about physical and sexual abuse in women's lives. No method of data collection, of course, can ensure that people will disclose sensitive information or be truthful is sharing their life course experiences all the time. But good ethnographic research—which is based on close-up, careful, and detailed observation; participation in the flow of activities with those being studied; and development of trust-based relationships—makes disclosure all the more likely.

In describing the processes involved in uncovering women's abuse experiences in the Three-City Study ethnography, we demonstrated the degree to which experiences of physical and sexual abuse permeate the lives of low-income mothers and present methodological and ethical challenges to ethnographers. Our process of uncovering abuse in women's lives was characterized by distinctive respondent disclosure patterns evoked by certain trigger topics, recent crisis events, and ethnographers' direct inquiries. The disclosure processes also involved ethnographers' own experiences with vicarious trauma and safety issues.

Because physical and sexual abuse often emerge naturalistically in ethnography and are rarely a starting point of inquiry, many ethnographic studies that uncover these issues may not, at the onset, address the consequent ethical and methodological considerations in the study design or planning. Like other studies, the Three-City Study principal investigators did not include extensive preplanning to address specifically the potential for participants' various patterns of disclosure and ethnographers' vicarious trauma. However, based on previous field experiences of the ethnographic study's director and several of the research staff, fieldworkers did receive training to address potential safety issues related to abuse prior to entering the field. Despite this precaution, the extent, amount, and intensity of respondent experiences were significantly greater than anticipated. Because the premise of the Three-City Study ethnography was based on the concept of structured discovery (Burton et al., 2005; Winston et al., 1999), these issues became a focus of inquiry, and comprehensive protocols to address a variety of ethical and methodological concerns were instituted immediately. Based on our experiences, we offer the following suggestions for practices to researchers that may be helpful in the process of uncovering physical and sexual abuse in studies of women's life course:

• Individuals who directly gather data from respondents should be provided with extensive training and supervision concerning physical and sexual abuse, potential disclosure patterns, and vicarious trauma before, during, and after work in the field. That training also should be extended to those who are analyzing data, even if they do not have direct contact with respondents. Some researchers may be concerned that a training emphasis on abuse experiences would likely introduce bias in researchers' interactions with respondents and in data analysts' interpretations of the data. Our experiences suggest that it is better for individuals to have a comprehensive understanding of these issues, and that the potential for bias in data gathering and analysis is actually minimized when researchers are better informed about the realities of abuse in women's lives and how uncovering that abuse may impact them as researchers.

- It is critical that principal investigators and interviewer supervisors occasionally accompany interviewers and ethnographers into the field to assess potential dangers and provide "second opinions" on observed family behaviors that appear troublesome. Joint observations and field experiences provide an important level of support to interviewers and ethnographers, and can move the "onus" for verifying and reporting abuse from those who gather data about the families directly to those who direct the studies. We also developed protocols about mandatory reporting of abuse that we reviewed and revised as needed.
- Developing site-specific lists of contacts for referrals to shelters and other support agencies is imperative for any study. Principal investigators, and interviewer and ethnographer supervisors, should also establish good working relationships with referring agencies and keep abreast of agencies' capacities to accommodate the needs of respondents should referrals take place.
- Any study that has the potential for uncovering abuse experiences should include research team members with clinical expertise in abuse, and make them available to staff and supervisors across the study for consultation. Having a "quick response" strategy in place to address ethnographers', interviewers', and data analysts' experiences with violence in the field, or with vicarious trauma, is also imperative. We put together a reporting and safety committee on the Three-City Study that comprised clinical psychologists, social workers, and lawyers who were able to convene in person or via conference call within 24 hours to address ethnographers' issues concerning abuse. We also scheduled periodic, project-wide conference calls devoted to issues of abuse, as well as local site team meetings to ensure consistent peer support and debriefing.

To our knowledge, none of the published literature from ethnographies that have explored domestic and sexual abuse addresses these methodological and ethical challenges or describes how the research staff addressed them in either planning or practice. The literature does indicate that sexual and domestic abuse are very likely to continue to emerge as issues in any ethnographic or intensive qualitative research conducted with women and families in low-income communities (e.g., Dodson, 1998; Edin, 2000; Edin & Kefalas, 2005; Fine & Weis, 1998; Kurz, 1996; Scott et al., 2002). And the use of intensive qualitative methods in the study of poverty in sociology and policy studies is likely to increase (Newman & Massengill, 2006). Given this, and based on our experiences in the Three-City Study ethnography, we argue that it is incumbent upon researchers engaged in inquiry in low-income communities to take issues of physical and sexual abuse into account in study design and planning. Particularly when studies involve the collection, analysis, and interpretation of narrative life course data, it is critical to address the ethical and methodological challenges posed by the potential development of vicarious trauma and issues of safety among all levels of project staff and informants.

ACKNOWLEDGMENTS

Writing and research for this chapter were supported by grants to Linda Burton from the National Science Foundation (No. SES 0703968) and the Administration on Children and Families (No. 90OJ2020), and core support to the Three-City Study from the National Institute of Child Health and Human Development through grant Nos. HD36093 and HD25936, as well as many other government agencies and private foundations. Most importantly, we thank the families who graciously participated in the research and who gave us access to their hidden life experiences.

REFERENCES

Abbott, A., & Hrycak, A. (1990). Measuring resemblance in sequence data. American Journal of Sociology, 96(1), 144–185.

Agar, M. H. (1996). The professional stranger: An informal introduction to ethnography. San Diego: Academic Press.

Allport, G. (1937). Personality: A psychological interpretation. New York: Holt.

Allport, G. W. (1954). The nature of prejudice. Reading, MA: Perseus.

Almeida, D. M. (2005). Resilience and vulnerability to daily stressors assessed via diary methods. Current Directions in Psychological Science, 14(2), 64–68.

Almeida, D. M., Chandler, A. L., & Wethington, E. (1999). Daily transmission of tensions between marital dyads and parent–child dyads. Journal of Marriage and the Family, 61(1), 49–61.

Almeida, D. M., & Horn, M. C. (2004). Is daily life more stressful during middle adulthood? In O. G. Brim, C. D. Ryff, & R. C. Kessler (Eds.), How healthy are we?: A national study of well-being at midlife (pp. 425–451). Chicago: University of Chicago Press.

Almeida, D. M., & Kessler, R. C. (1998). Everyday stressors and gender differences in daily distress. Journal of Personality and Social Psychology, 75(3), 670–680.

Almeida, D. M., Serido, J., & McDonald, D. (2006). Daily life stressors of early and late Baby Boomers. In S. K. Whitbourne & S. L. Willis (Eds.), The Baby Boomers grow up: Contemporary perspectives on midlife (pp. 165–184). Mahwah, NJ: Erlbaum.

Almeida, D. M., Wethington, E., & Kessler, R. C. (2002). The Daily Inventory of Stressful Experiences (DISE): An interview-based approach for measuring daily stressors. Assessment, 9 (1), 41–55.

Alter, G., & Oris, M. (2001). The family and mortality: A case study from rural Belgium. Annales de Dèmographie Historique, 101, 11–31.

Altobelli, J., & Moen, P. (2007). Work–family spillover among dual-earner couples. In J. J. Suitor & T. J. Owens (Eds.), Advances in life course research: Interpersonal relations across the life course (Vol. 12, pp. 361–382). Oxford, England: Elsevier Science.

Altucher, K., & Williams, L. B. (2003). Family clocks: Timing parenthood. In P. Moen (Ed.), It's about time: Couples and careers (pp. 49–59). Ithaca, N Y: Cornell University Press.

Amato, P. R., & Booth, A. (2001). The legacy of parents' marital discord: Consequences for children's marital quality. Journal of Personality and Social Psychology, 81(4), 627–638.

Anderson, C. A., Bowman, M. J., & Tinto, V. (1972). Where colleges are and who attends: Effects of accessibility on college attendance. New York: McGraw-Hill.

Andersson, F., Holzer, H. J., & Lane, J. I. (2005). Moving up or moving on: Who advances in the low-wage labor market? New York: Russell Sage Foundation.

Andrew, M., & Hauser, R. M. (2008, August). Evaluating the "strategic center": Race–ethnic differences in updating and applying educational expectations. Paper presented at the annual meeting of the American Sociological Association, Boston, MA.

Aneshensel, C. S., Botticello, A. L., & Yamamoto-Mitani, N. (2004). When caregiving ends: The course of depressive symptoms after bereavement. Journal of Health and Social Behavior, 45(3), 422–440.

Antonucci, T. C., & Akiyama, H. (1995). Convoys of social relations: Family and friendships within a life span context. In R. Blieszner & V. H. Bedford (Eds.), Handbook of aging and the family (pp. 355–371). Westport, CT: Greenwood Press.

Asher, R. M., & Fine, G. A. (1991). Fragile ties: Shaping relationships with women married to alcoholics. In W. B. Shaffir & R. A. Stebbins (Eds.), Experiencing fieldwork: An inside view of qualitative research (pp. 196–205). Newbury Park, CA: Sage.

Atwood, N. C. (2007). Growing up bookish in a working class world. Manuscript under review.

Bachman, R., & Saltzman, L. E. (1995). Violence against women: Estimates from the redesigned survey. Washington, DC: Bureau of Justice Statistics.

Baltes, P. B. (1987). Theoretical propositions of life-span developmental psychology: On the dynamics between growth and decline. Developmental Psychology, 23(5), 611–626.

Baltes, P. B., & Baltes, M. M. (1990). Psychological perspectives on successful aging: The model of selective optimization with compensation. In Successful aging: Perspectives from the behavioral sciences (pp. 1–34). Cambridge, England: Cambridge University Press.

Baltrus, P. T., Lynch, J. W., Everson-Rose, S., Raghunathan, T. E., & Kaplan, G. A. (2005). Race/ethnicity, life course socioeconomic position, and body weight trajectories over 34 years: The Alameda County Study. American Journal of Public Health, 95(9), 1595–1601.

Barker, D. J. P. (2001). Fetal origins of cardiovascular and lung disease. New York: Dekker.

Barrett, A. E. (2000). Marital trajectories and mental health. Journal of Health and Social Behavior, 41, 451–464.

Bauer, D., & Curran, P. J. (2003). Distributional assumptions of growth mixture models: Implications for over-extraction of latent trajectory classes. Psychological Methods, 8 (3), 338–363.

Beck, U. (1992). Risk society: Towards a new modernity. London: Sage.

Becker, G. S. (1981). A treatise on the family. Cambridge, MA: Harvard University Press.

Becker, H. S. (1960). Notes on the concept of commitment. American Journal of Sociology, 66(1), 32–40.

Becker, H. S. (1996). The epistemology of qualitative research. In R. Jessor, A. Colby, & R. A. Shweder (Eds.), Ethnography and human development: Context and meaning in social inquiry (pp. 53–71). Chicago: University of Chicago Press.

Becker, P. E., & Moen, P. (1999). Scaling back: Dual-career couples' work–family strategies. Journal of Marriage and the Family, 61(3), 995–1007.

Becker-Blease, K. A., & Freyd, J. J. (2006). Research participants telling the truth about their lives: The ethics of asking and not asking about abuse. American Psychologist, 61(3), 218–226.

Benedict, R. (1946). The chrysanthemum and the sword: Patterns of Japanese culture. Boston: Houghton Mifflin.

Bengston, V. L. (1975). Generation and family effects in value socialization. American Sociological Review, 40 (3), 358–371.

Bengston, V. L. (2001). Beyond the nuclear family: The increasing importance of multigenerational bonds. Journal of Marriage and the Family, 63(1), 1–16.

Bennett, J. B., & Lehman, W. E. (1999). Employee exposure to coworker substance use and negative consequences: The moderating effects of work group membership. Journal of Health and Social Behavior, 40 (2), 307–322.

Bernhardt, A., Morris, M., Handcock, M. S., & Scott, M. A. (2001). Divergent paths: Economic mobility in the new American labor market. New York: Sage.

Bertaux, D. (1981). Life stories in the bakers' trade. In D. Bertaux & I. BertauxWiame (Eds.), Biography and society: The life history approach in the social sciences (pp. 169–189). Beverly Hills, CA: Sage.

Bertaux, D., & Bertaux-Wiame, I. (Eds.). Biography and society: The life history approach in the social sciences. Beverly Hills, CA: Sage.

Bertaux, D., & Kohli, M. (1984). The life story approach: A continental view. Annual Review of Sociology, 10, 215–237.

Bertaux, D., & Thompson, P. (1997). Pathways to social class: A qualitative approach to social mobility. New York: Oxford University Press.

Bertaux-Wiame, I. (1981). The life history approach to the study of internal migration. In D. Bertaux & I. Bertaux-Wiame(Eds.), Biography and society: The life history approach in the social sciences (pp. 249–265). Beverly Hills, CA: Sage.

Bianchi, S. M., Robinson, J. P., & Milkie, M. A. (2006). Changing rhythms of American family life. New York: Russell Sage Foundation.

Bielby, D. D., & Bielby, W. T. (1988). She works hard for the money: Household responsibilities and the allocation of work effort. American Journal of Sociology, 93(5), 1031–1059.

Bielby, W. T., & Hauser, R. M. (1977). Response error in earnings functions for nonblack males. Sociological Methods and Research, 6(2), 241–280.

Bielby, W. T., Hauser, R. M., & Featherman, D. L. (1977). Response errors of black and nonblack males in models of the intergenerational transmission of socioeconomic status. American Journal of Sociology, 82(6), 1242–1288.

Bilgrad, R. (1990). National Death Index user's manual. Hyattsville, MD: U.S. Department of Health and Human Services, Public Health Service, Centers for Disease Control, National Center for Health Statistics.

Birch, M., & Miller, T. (2000). Inviting intimacy: The interview as therapeutic opportunity. International Journal of Social Research Methodology, 3 (3), 189–202.

Birdett, K. S., Fingerman, K. L., & Almeida, D. M. (2005). Age differences in exposure and reactions to interpersonal tensions: A daily diary study. Psychology and Aging, 20 (2), 330–340.

Blair-Loy, M. (1999). Career patterns of executive women in finance: An optimal matching analysis. American Journal of Sociology, 104(4), 1346–1397.

Blair-Loy, M., & Wharton, A. S. (2002). Employees' use of work–family policies and the workplace social context. Social Forces, 80 (3), 813–845.

Blanchard-Fields, F., & Cooper, C. (2004). Social cognition and social relationships. In F. R. Lang & K. L. Fingerman (Eds.), Growing together: Personal relationships across the lifespan (pp. 268–289). New York: Cambridge University Press.

Blatter, C. W., & Jacobsen, J. J. (1993). Older women coping with divorce: Peer support groups. Women and Therapy, 14(1/2), 141–155.

Blau, P.M. (1994). Structural contexts of opportunities. Chicago: University of Chicago Press.

Blau, P.M., & Duncan, O.D. (1967). The American occupational structure. New York: Wiley.

Blossfeld, H.-P. (1986). Career opportunities in the Federal Republic of Germany: A dynamic approach to the study of life course, cohort, and period effects. European Sociological Review, 2 (3), 208–225.

Blossfeld, H.-P. (1995). The new role of women. Family formation in modern societies. Boulder, CO: Westview Press.

Blossfeld, H.-P., Buchholz, S., & Hofäcker, D. (2006). Globalization, uncertainty and late careers in society. New York: Routledge.

Blossfeld, H.-P., DeRose, A., Hoem, J.M., & Rohwer, G. (1995). Education, modernization, and the risk of marriage disruption: Differences in the effect of women's educational attainment in Sweden, West Germany, and Italy. In K.O. Mason & A.-M. Jenson (Eds.), Gender and family change in industrialized countries (pp. 200–222). Oxford, England: Clarendon.

Blossfeld, H.-P., & Drobnič, S. (2001). Careers of couples in contemporary societies. From male breadwinner to dual-earner families. Oxford, England: Oxford University Press.

Blossfeld, H.-P., Golsch, K., & Rohwer, G. (2007). Event history analysis with Stata. Mahwah, NJ: Erlbaum.

Blossfeld, H.-P., & Hakim, C. (1997). Between equalization and marginalization: Women working part-time in Europe and the United States of America. Oxford, England: Oxford University Press.

Blossfeld, H.-P., & Hofmeister, H.A.E. (2006). Globalization, uncertainty and women's careers in international comparison. Cheltenham, England: Edward Elgar.

Blossfeld, H.-P., & Huinink, J. (1991). Human capital investments or norms of role transition?: How women's schooling and career affect the process of family formation. American Journal of Sociology, 97(1), 143–168.

Blossfeld, H.-P., & Mayer, K.U. (1988). Labor market segmentation in the FRG: An empirical study of segmentation theories from a life course perspective. European Sociological Review, 4(2), 123–140.

Blossfeld, H.-P., & Mills, M. (2001). A causal approach to interrelated family events: A cross-national comparison of cohabitation, nonmarital conception, and marriage. Canadian Journal of Population, 28 (2), 409–437.

Blossfeld, H.-P., Mills, M., & Bernardi, F.E. (2006). Globalization, uncertainty and men's careers in international comparison. Cheltenham, England: Edward Elgar.

Blossfeld, H.-P., Mills, M., K lijzing, E., & Kurz, K.E. (2005). Globalization, uncertainty and youth in society. London: Routledge.

Blossfeld, H.-P., & Stockmann, R. (1998/1999). Globalization and changes in vocational training systems in developing and advanced industrialized societies, Vol. I–III. International Journal of Sociology, 28 (4), 29 (1, 2).

Blossfeld, H.-P., & Timm, A. (2003). Who marries whom?: Educational systems as marriage markets in modern societies. Dordrecht: K luwer Academic.

Blumer, H. (1955). Attitudes and the social act. Social Problems, 3(2), 59–65. Blumstein, A., Cohen, J., & Farrington, D.P. (1988a). Criminal career research: Its value for criminology. Criminology, 26(1), 1–35.

Blumstein, A., Cohen, J., & Farrington, D.P. (1988b). Longitudinal and criminal career research: Further clarifications. Criminology, 26(1), 57–74. Blumstein, A., Cohen, J., Roth, J.A., & Visher, C. (Eds.). (1986). Criminal careers and career criminals. Washington, DC: National Academies Press.

Blyth, D.A., Simmons, R.G., & Carlton-Ford, S. (1983). The adjustment of early adolescents to school transitions. Journal of Early Adolescence, 31(1–2), 105–120.

Boardman, J.D. (2009). State-level moderation of genetic tendencies to smoke cigarettes. American Journal of Public Health, 99 (3), 480–486.

Boardman, J.D., Saint Onge, J.M., Haberstick, B.C., Timberlake, D.S., & Hewitt, J.K. (2008). Do schools moderate the genetic determinants of smoking? Behavior Genetics, 38 (3), 234–246.

Bolger, N., Davis, A., & Rafaeli, E. (2003). Diary methods: Capturing life as it is lived. Annual Review of Psychology, 54, 579–616.

Bolger, N., DeLongis, A., Kessler, R.C., & Schilling, E. (1989). Effects of daily stress on negative mood. Journal of Personality and Social Psychology, 57(5), 808–818.

Bowles, S. (1972). Schooling and inequality from generation to generation. Journal of Political Economy, 80 (3), S219–S251.

Breen, R. (1997). Risk recommodification and the future of the service class. Sociology, 31(3), 473–489.

Bride, B.E. (2007). Prevalence of secondary traumatic stress among social workers. Social Work, 52 (1), 63–70.

Brim, O.G. (1992). Ambition: How we manage success and failure throughout our lives. New York: Basic Books.

Brim, O.G., Jr., & Ryff, C. (1980). On the properties of life events. In P.G. Baltes & O.G. Brim (Eds.), Life-span development and behavior (Vol. 3, pp. 368–388). New York: Academic Press.

Brines, J. (1994). Economic dependency, gender, and division of labor at home. American Journal of Sociology, 100 (2), 652–688.

Brines, J., & Joyner, K. (1999). The ties that bind: Principles of cohesion in cohabitation and marriage. American Sociological Review, 64(2), 333–355.

Bronfenbrenner, U., & Ceci, S.J. (1994). Nature–nurture reconceptualized in developmental perspective: A bioecological model. Psychological Review, 101(4), 568–586.

Bronfenbrenner, U., & Crouter, A.C. (1983). The evolution of environmental models in developmental research. In P.H. Mussen (Ed.), Handbook of child psychology: Vol. 1. History, theory, and methods (pp. 357–414). New York: Wiley.

Brown, G., & Harris, T. (1978). Social origins of depression: A study of psychiatric disorder in women. New York: Free Press.

Brown, G.W., & Harris, T.O. (1989). Life events and illness. New York: Guilford Press.

Brown, L.M., & Gilligan, C. (1992). Meeting at the crossroads: Women's psychology and girls' development. Cambridge, MA: Harvard University Press.

Brown, T.H. (2008). Divergent pathways: Racial/ethnic inequalities in wealth and health trajectories. PhD dissertation, University of North Carolina at Chapel Hill.

Brückner, E., & Mayer, K.U. (1998). Collecting life history data: Experiences from the German life history study. In J.Z. Giele & G.H. Elder, Jr. (Eds.), Methods of life course research: Qualitative and quantitative approaches (pp. 152–181). Thousand Oaks, CA: Sage.

Bryk, A.S., & Raudenbush, S.W. (1992). Hierarchical linear models: Applications and data analysis methods (Vol. 1). Newbury Park, CA: Sage.

Buchmann, M. (1989). The script of life in modern society: Entry into adulthood in a changing world. Chicago: University of Chicago Press.

Burke, K. (1945). A grammar of motives. New York: Prentice-Hall.

Burks, B.S., Jensen, D.W., & Terman, L.M. (1959). Follow-up studies of a thousand gifted children. Stanford, CA: Stanford University Press.

Burton, L.M. (1990). Teenage childbearing as an alternative life-course strategy in multigeneration black families. Human Nature, 1(2), 123–143.

Burton, L.M. (1996). Age norms, the timing of family role transitions, and intergenerational caregiving among aging African American women. Gerontologist, 36(2), 199–208.

Burton, L.M. (1997). Ethnography and the meaning of adolescence in highrisk neighborhoods. Ethos, 25(1), 208–217.

Burton, L.M., Cherlin, A., Winn, D.M., Estacion, A., & Holder-Taylor, C. (in press). The role of trust in low-income mothers' intimate unions. Journal of Marriage and Family.

Burton, L.M., Obeidallah, D.A., & Allison, K. (1996). Ethnographic insights on social context and adolescent development among inner-city AfricanAmerican teens. In R. Jessor, A. Colby, & R. Shweder (Eds.), Ethnography and human development: Context and meaning in social inquiry (pp. 395–418). Chicago: University of Chicago Press.

Burton, L.M., Skinner, D., & Matthews, S. (2005, August). "Structuring discovery": A model and method for multi-site team ethnography. Paper presented at the annual meeting of the American Sociological Association, Philadelphia, PA.

Butler, J., & Burton, L.M. (1990). Rethinking teenage childbearing: Is sexual abuse a missing link? Family Relations, 39 (1), 73–80.

Button, T.M.M., Corley, R.P., Rhee, S.H., Hewitt, J.K., Young, S.E., & Stallings, M.C. (2007). Delinquent peer affiliation and conduct problems: A twin study. Journal of Abnormal Psychology, 116(3), 554–564.

Butz, W.P., & Torrey, B.B. (2006). Some frontiers in social science. Science, 312(5782), 1898–1900.

Cadoret, R.J., Yates, W.R., Troughton, E., Woodworth, G., & Stewart, M. (1995). Genetic–environmental interaction in the genesis of aggressivity and conduct disorders. Archives of General Psychiatry, 52 (11), 916–924.

Cameron, S.J., Armstrong-Stassen, M., Orr, R.R., & Loukas, A. (1991). Stress, coping, and resources in mothers of adults with developmental disabilities. Counseling Psychology Quarterly, 4(4), 301–310.

Campbell, R.T., & Henretta, J.C. (1980). Status claims and status attainment: The determinants of financial well-being. American Journal of Sociology, 86(3), 618–629.

Carstensen, L.L., Isaacowitz, D.M., & Charles, S.T. (1999). Taking time seriously: A theory of socioemotional selectivity. American Psychologist, 54(3), 165–181.

Caspi, A. (2004). Life-course development: The interplay of social selection and social causation within and across generations. In P.L. Chase-Lansdale, K. K iernan, & R.J. Friedman (Eds.), Human development across lives and generations: The potential for change. New York: Cambridge University Press.

Caspi, A., & Moffitt, T.E. (1993). When do individual differences matter?: A paradoxical theory of personality coherence. Psychological Inquiry, 4(4), 247–271.

Caspi, A., Moffitt, T.E., Mill, J., Martin, J., Craig, I.W., Taylor, A., et al. (2002). Role of genotype in the cycle of violence in maltreated children. Science, 297(5582), 851–854.

Caspi, A., Sugden, K., Moffitt, T.E., Taylor, A., Craig, I.W., Harrington, H., et al. (2003). Influence of life stress on depression: Moderation in the 5 -HTT gene. Science, 301(5631), 386–389.

Cassell, J., & Wax, M.L. (1980). Toward a moral science of human beings. Social Problems, 27(3), 259–264.

Cherlin, A.J., Burton, L.M., Hurt, T.R., & Purvin, D.M. (2004). The influence of physical and sexual abuse on marriage and cohabitation. American Sociological Review, 69 (6), 768–789.

Chesley, N. (2005). Blurring boundaries?: Linking technology use, spillover, individual distress, and family satisfaction. Journal of Marriage and the Family, 67(5), 1237–1248.

Chesley, N., & Moen, P. (2006). When workers care: Dual-earner couples' caregiving strategies benefit use, and psychological well-being. American Behavioral Scientist, 49 (9), 1–22.

Chiriboga, D. A. (1989). Stress and loss in middle age. In R. A. Kalish (Ed.), Midlife loss: Coping strategies (pp. 42–88). Thousand Oaks, CA: Sage. Chiriboga, D. A. (1997). Crisis, challenge, and stability in the middle years. In M. E. Lachman & J. B. James (Eds.), Multiple paths of midlife development (pp. 293–322). Chicago: University of Chicago Press.

Christakis, N. A., & Fowler, J. H. (2007). The spread of obesity in a large social network over 32 years. New England Journal of Medicine, 357(4), 370–379.

Chung, I.-J., Hill, K. G., Hawkins, J. D., Gilchrist, L. D., & Nagin, D. S. (2002). Childhood predictors of offense trajectories. Journal of Research in Crime and Delinquency, 39 (1), 60–90.

Clark, L. A., & Watson, D. (1988). Mood and the mundane: Relations between daily life events and self-reported mood. Journal of Personality and Social Psychology, 54(2), 296–308.

Clarkberg, M. (1999). The price of partnering: The role of economic well-being in young adults' first union experiences. Social Forces, 77(3), 945–968. Clarkberg, M., & Moen, P. (2001). Understanding the time-squeeze: Married couples preferred and actual work-hour strategies. American Behavioral Scientist, 44(7), 1115–1136.

Clarke, M. (1975). Survival in the field: Implications of personal experience in fieldwork. Theory and Society, 2 (1), 95–123.

Clark-Plaskie, M., & Lachman, M. E. (1999). The sense of control in midlife. In S. L. Willis & J. D. Reid (Eds.), Life in the middle: Psychological and social development in middle age (pp. 181–208). San Diego: Academic Press.

Clarridge, B. R., Sheehy, L. L., & Hauser, T. S. (1977). Tracing members of a panel: A 17-year follow-up. In K. F. Schuessler (Ed.), Sociological methodology 1978 (pp. 185–203). San Francisco: Jossey-Bass.

Clausen, J. A. (1986). The life course: A sociological perspective. Englewood Cliffs, NJ: Prentice-Hall.

Clausen, J. A. (1991). Adolescent competence and the shaping of the life course. American Journal of Sociology, 96(4), 805–842.

Clausen, J. A. (1993). American lives: Looking back at the children of the Great Depression. New York: Free Press.

Clipp, E. C., Pavalko, E. K., & Elder, G. H., Jr. (1992). Trajectories of health: In concept and empirical pattern. Behavior, Health, and Aging, 2(3), 159–179.

Coard, S. J., & Sellers, R. M. (2005). African American families as a context for racial socialization. In V. C. Lloyd, N. E. Hill, & K. A. Dodge (Eds.), African American family life (pp. 264–284). New York: Guilford Press.

Cohen, S., Kessler, R. C., & Gordon, L. U. (1997). Strategies for measuring stress in studies of psychiatric and physical disorders. In S. Cohen, R. C. Kessler, & L. U. Gordon (Eds.), Measuring stress: A guide for health and social scientists (pp. 3–26). New York: Oxford University Press.

Coleman, J. S., with the assistance of Johnstone, J. W. C., & Jonassohn, K. (1961). The adolescent society: The social life of the teenager and its impact on education. New York: Free Press of Glencoe.

Coleman, J. S. (1981). Longitudinal data analysis. New York: Basic Books. Collins, L. M. (2006). Analysis of longitudinal data: The integration of theoretical model, temporal design, and statistical model. Annual Review of Psychology, 57, 505–528.

Coltrane, S. (1996). Family man: Fatherhood, housework, and gender equity. New York: Oxford University Press.

Coltrane, S., & Adams, M. (2001). Men's family work: Child-centered fathering and the sharing of domestic labor. In R. Hertz & N. L. Marshall (Eds.), Working families: The transformation of the American home (pp. 72–99). Berkeley: University of California Press.

Connell, R.W. (1995). Masculinities. Berkeley: University of California Press.

Courgeau, D., & Lelièvre, E. (1992). Event history analysis in demography. Oxford, England: Clarendon.

Cowan, C.P., & Cowan, P.G. (1999). When partners become parents: The big life change for couples. Mahwah, NJ: Erlbaum.

Cross, S., & Markus, H. (1991). Possible selves across the life span. Human Development, 34(4), 230–255.

Croudace, T.J., Jarvelin, M.-R., Wadsworth, M.E.J., & Jones, P.B. (2003). Developmental typology of trajectories of nighttime bladder control: Epidemiologic application of longitudinal latent class analysis. American Journal of Epidemiology, 157(9), 834–842.

Crowder, K., & South, S.J. (2008). Spatial dynamics of white flight: The effects of local and extralocal racial conditions on neighborhood out-migration. American Sociological Review, 73(5), 792–812.

Crystal, S., & Waehrer, K. (1996). Later life economic inequality in longitudinal perspective. Journals of Gerontology B: Psychological Sciences and Social Sciences, 51(6), S307–S318.

Csikszentmihalyi, M. (1993). The evolving self: A psychology for the third millenium. New York: HarperCollins.

Csikszentmihalyi, M., & Beattie, O. (1979). Life themes: A theoretical and empirical exploration of their origins and effects. Journal of Humanistic Psychology, 19, 45–63.

Cudeck, R., & K lebe, K.J. (2002). Multiphase mixed-effects models for repeated measures data. Psychological Methods, 7(1), 41–63.

Curran, P.J., & Willoughby, M.T. (2003). Implications of latent trajectory models for the study of developmental psychopathology. Development and Psychopathology, 15(3), 581–612.

Dahlin, E., Kelly, E., & Moen, P. (2008). Is work the new neighborhood?: Social ties in the workplace, family, and neighborhood. Sociological Quarterly, 49 (4), 719–736.

Daly, K. (2003). Family theory versus the theories families live by. Journal of Marriage and the Family, 65(4), 771–784.

Dannefer, D. (1987). Aging as intracohort differentiation: Accentuation, the Matthew effect, and the life course. Sociological Forum, 2(2), 211–236.

Dannefer, D. (2003). Cumulative advantage/disadvantage and the life course: Cross fertilizing age and social science theory. Journals of Gerontology B: Psychological Sciences and Social Sciences, 58 (6), S327–S338.

Dannefer, D., & Sell, R.R. (1988). Age structure, the life course, and "aged heterogeneity." Contemporary Sociology, 2(1), 1–10.

Davis, J.A., & Smith, T.W. (1992). The NORC General Social Survey: A user's guide. Newbury Park, CA: Sage.

Dean, J.P., & Williams, R.M. (1956). Social and cultural factors affecting role conflict and adjustment among American women: A pilot investigation. Bethesda, MD: National Institute of Mental Health.

Dempster-McClain, D., & Moen, P. (1997). Finding respondents in a follow-up study. In J.Z. Giele & G.H. Elder, Jr. (Eds.), Methods of life course research (pp. 128–151). Thousand Oaks, CA: Sage.

Dentinger, E., & Clarkberg, M. (2002). Informal caregiving and retirement timing among men and women: Gender and caregiving relationships in late midlife. Journal of Family Issues, 23(7), 857–879.

Deutscher, I. (1966). Words and deeds: Social science and social policy. Social Problems, 13(3), 235–254.

Dick, D.M., Agrawal, A., Schuckit, M.A., Bierut, L., Hinrichs, A., Fox, L., et al. (2006). Marital status, alcohol dependence, and GABR A2: Evidence for gene–environment correlation and interaction. Journal of Studies on Alcohol, 67(2), 185–194.

Dillman, D.A. (1991). The design and administration of mail surveys. Annual Review of Sociology, 17, 225–249.

Dillman, D.A. (2000). Mail and Internet surveys: The tailored design method. New York: Wiley.

Dillon, M., & Wink, P. (2007). In the course of a lifetime: Tracing religious belief, practice, and change. Berkeley: University of California Press.

DiPrete, T.A., de Graaf, P.M., Luijkx, R., Tåhlin, M., & Blossfeld, H.-P. (1997). Collectivist versus Individualist Mobility Regimes?: Structural change and job mobility in four countries. American Journal of Sociology, 103(2), 318–358.

DiPrete, T.A., & Eirich, G.M. (2006). Cumulative advantage as a mechanism for inequality: A review of theoretical and empirical developments. Annual Review of Sociology, 32, 271–297.

Dodson, L. (1998). Don't call us out of name: The untold lives of women and girls in poor America. Boston: Beacon Press.

Dodson, L., & Schmalzbauer, L. (2005). Poor mothers and habits of hiding: Participatory methods in poverty research. Journal of Marriage and Family, 67(4), 949–959.

Dohrenwend, B.S., & Dohrenwend, B.P. (1974). Stressful life events: Their nature and effects. New York: Wiley-Interscience.

D'Onofrio, B.M., Turkheimer, E., Emery, R.E., Slutske, W.S., Heath, A.C., Madden, P.A., et al. (2005). A genetically informed study of marital instability and its association with offspring psychopathology. Journal of Abnormal Psychology, 114(4), 570–586.

Drobnic, S., & Blossfeld, H.-P. (2004). Career patterns over the life course: Gender, class, and linked lives. In A.L. Kalleberg, S.L. Morgan, J. Myles, & R.A. Rosenfeld (Eds.), Inequality: Structures, dynamics and mechanisms: Essays in honor of Aage B. Sørensen (Vol. 21, pp. 139–164). Amsterdam: Elsevier.

Dumais, S.A. (2002). The educational pathways of white working-class students. Unpublished PhD dissertation, Harvard University, Cambridge, MA. Duncan, G.J., & Morgan, J.N. (1985). The panel study of income dynamics. In G.H. Elder, Jr. (Ed.), Life course dynamics: Trajectories and transitions: 1968–1980 (pp. 50–71). Ithaca, N Y: Cornell University Press.

Duncan, O.D. (1968). Ability and achievement. Eugenics Quarterly, 15(1), 1–11. Duneier, M. (2007). On the legacy of Elliot Liebow and Carol Stack: Context-driven fieldwork and the need for continuous ethnography. Focus, 25(1), 33–38.

D'Unger, A.V., Land, K.C., McCall, P.L., & Nagin, D.S. (1998). How many latent classes of delinquent/criminal careers?: Results from mixed Poisson regression analyses. American Journal of Sociology, 103(6), 1593–1630.

Dunn, K.M., Jordan, K., & Croft, P.S. (2006). Characterizing the course of low back pain: A latent class analysis. American Journal of Epidemiology, 163(8), 754–761.

Easterlin, R.A. (1987). Birth and fortune: The impact of numbers on personal welfare (2nd ed.). Chicago: University of Chicago Press.

Eccles, J.S., & Midgley, C. (1989). Stage–environment fit: Developmentally appropriate classrooms for early adolescents. In R.E. Ames & C. Ames (Eds.), Research on motivation in education (Vol. 3, pp. 139–186). New York: Academic Press.

Edin, K. (2000). What do low-income single mothers say about marriage? Social Problems, 47(1), 112–133.

Edin, K., & Kefalas, M. (2005). Promises I can keep: Why poor women put motherhood before marriage. Berkeley: University of California Press.

Eggleston, E.P., Laub, J.H., & Sampson, R.J. (2004). Methodological sensitivities to latent class analysis of long-term criminal trajectories. Journal of Quantitative Criminology, 20 (1), 1–26.

Eichorn, D.H., Clausen, J.A., Haan, N., Honzik, M.P., & Mussen, P.H. (1981). Present and past in middle life. New York: Academic Press.

Elder, G.H., Jr. (Ed.). (1973). Linking social structure and personality. Beverly Hills, CA: Sage.

Elder, G.H., Jr. (1974). Children of the Great Depression: Social change in life experience. Chicago: University of Chicago Press.

Elder, G.H., Jr. (1975). Age differentiation and the life course. Annual Review of Sociology, 1, 165–190.

Elder, G.H., Jr. (Ed.). (1985a). Life course dynamics: Trajectories and transitions, 1968–1980. Ithaca, N Y: Cornell University Press.

Elder, G.H., Jr. (1985b). Perspectives on the life course. In Life course dynamics: Trajectories and transitions, 1968–1980 (pp. 23–49). Ithaca, N Y: Cornell University Press.

Elder, G.H., Jr. (1986). Military times and turning points in men's lives. Developmental Psychology, 22 (2), 233–245.

Elder, G.H., Jr. (1987a). Familes and lives: Some developments in life-course studies. Journal of Family History, 12, 179–199.

Elder, G.H., Jr. (1987b). War mobilization and the life course: A cohort of World War II veterans. Sociological Forum, 2 (3), 449–472.

Elder, G.H., Jr. (1994). Time, human agency, and social change: Perspectives on the life course. Social Psychology Quarterly, 57(1), 4–15.

Elder, G.H., Jr. (1998a). The life course as developmental theory. Child Development, 69 (1), 1–12.

Elder, G.H., Jr. (1998b). The life course and human development. In R.M. Lerner (Ed.), Handbook of child psychology (5th ed.): Vol. 1. Theoretical models of human development (pp. 939–991). New York: Wiley.

Elder, G.H., Jr. (1999). Children of the Great Depression: Social change in life experience (25th anniversary edition). Boulder, CO: Westview Press.

Elder, G.H., Jr. (2000). Life course theory. In A.E. Kazdin (Ed.), Encyclopedia of psychology (3rd ed., Vol. 5, pp. 50–52). Washington, DC: American Psychological Association.

Elder, G.H., Jr., & Clipp, E.C. (1988). Wartime losses and social bonding: Influences across 40 years in men's lives. Psychiatry, 51, 177–198.

Elder, G.H., Jr., & Conger, R.D. (2000). Legacies of the land. In G.H. Elder, Jr. & R.D. Conger (Eds.), Children of the land: Adversity and success in rural America (pp. 221–249). Chicago: University of Chicago Press.

Elder, G.H., Jr., George, L.K., & Shanahan, M.J. (1996). Psychosocial stress over the life course. In H. Kaplan (Ed.), Psychosocial stress: Perspective on structure, theory, life-course, and methods (pp. 247–292). San Diego: Academic Press.

Elder, G.H., Jr., Johnson, M.K., & Crosnoe, R. (2003). The emergence and development of the life course. In J.T. Mortimer & M.J. Shanahan (Eds.), Handbook of the life course. New York: Plenum Press.

Elder, G.H., Jr., & O'Rand, A.M. (1995). Adult lives in a changing society. In K.S. Cook, G.A. Fine, & J.S. House (Eds.), Sociological perspectives on social psychology (pp. 452–475). Boston: Allyn & Bacon.

Elder, G.H., Jr., Pavalko, E.K., & Clipp, E.C. (1993). Working with archival data: Studying lives (Vol. 07088). Newbury Park, CA: Sage.

Elder, G.H., Jr., & Rockwell, R.C. (1979a). Economic depression and postwar opportunity in men's lives: A study of life patterns and health. Research in Community and Mental Health, 1, 249–303.

Elder, G.H., Jr., & Rockwell, R.C. (1979b). The life-course and human development: An ecological perspective. International Journal of Behavioral Development, 2, 1–21.

Elder, G.H., Jr., & Shanahan, M.J. (2006). The life course and human development. In R.E. Lerner (Ed.), Handbook of child psychology (6th ed., Vol. 1, pp. 665–715). Hoboken, NJ: Wiley.

Elder, G.H., Jr., Shanahan, M.J., & Clipp, E.C. (1994). When war comes to men's lives: Life course patterns in family, work, and health. Psychology and Aging, 9 (1), 5–16.

Elder, G.H., Jr., Shanahan, M.J., & Clipp, E.C. (1997). Linking combat and physical health: The legacy of World War II in men's lives. American Journal of Psychiatry, 154(3), 330–336.

Elliott, M.R., Shope, J.T., Raghunathan, T.E., & Waller, P.F. (2006). Gender differences among young drivers in the association between high-risk driving and substance use/environmental influences. Journal of Studies on Alcohol, 67(2), 252–260.

Elman, C., & O'Rand, A.M. (1998). Midlife entry into vocational training: A mobility model. Social Science Research, 27, 128–158.

Elman, C., & O'Rand, A.M. (2002). Perceived labor market insecurity and entry into work-related education and training among adult workers. Social Science Research, 31, 49–76.

Elman, C., & O'Rand, A.M. (2004). The race is to the swift: Socioeconomic origins, adult education, and wage attainment. American Journal of Sociology, 110 (1), 123–160.

Elman, C., & O'Rand, A.M. (2007). The effects of social origins, life events, and institutional sorting on adults' school transitions. Social Science Research, 36(3), 1276–1299.

Elo, I.T., & Preston, S.H. (1996). Educational differentials in mortality: United States, 1979–85. Social Science and Medicine, 42 (1), 47–57.

Elo, I.T., Turra, C.M., Kestenbaum, B., & Ferguson, B.R. (2004). Mortality among elderly Hispanics in the United States: Past evidence and new results. Demography, 41(1), 109–128.

Emerson, R.M., & Pollner, M. (2001). Constructing participant–observation relations. In R.M. Emerson & M. Pollner (Eds.), Contemporary field research: Perspectives and formulations (pp. 239–259). Prospect Heights, IL: Waveland Press.

Erikson, E.H. (1963). Childhood and society (2nd ed.). New York: Norton.

Erikson, R., & Jonsson, J.O. (1996). Can education be equalized?: The Swedish case in comparative perspective. Boulder, CO: Westview Press.

Esping-Andersen, G. (1990). The three worlds of welfare capitalism. Cambridge, England: Polity Press.

Etherington, K. (2007). Working with traumatic stories: From transcriber to witness. International Journal of Social Research Methodology, 10 (2), 85–97.

Featherman, D.L., & Hauser, R.M. (1975). Design for a replicate study of social mobility in the United States. In K.C. Land & S.S. Spilerman (Eds.), Social indicator models (pp. 219–251). New York: Russell Sage Foundation.

Featherman, D.L., & Hauser, R.M. (1978). Opportunity and change. New York: Academic Press.

Feerick, M.M., & Haugaard, J.J. (1999). Long-term effects of witnessing marital violence for women: The contribution of childhood physical and sexual abuse. Journal of Family Violence, 14(4), 377–398.

Feng, D., Silverstein, M., Giarrusso, R., McArdle, J.J., & Bengston, V.L. (2006). Attrition of older adults in longitudinal surveys: Detection and correction of sample selection bias using multigenerational data. Journals of Gerontology B: Psychological Sciences and Social Sciences, 61(6), S323–S328.

Fergusson, D.M., Horwood, L.J., & Nagin, D.S. (2000). Offending trajectories in a New Zealand birth cohort. Criminology, 38(2), 525–551.

Ferraro, K. F., & Kelley-Moore, J. A. (2003). Cumulative disadvantage and health: Long-term consequences of obesity? American Sociological Review, 68 (5), 707–729.

Ferri, E., Bynner, J., & Wadsworth, M. (Eds.). (2003). Changing Britain, changing lives: Three generations at the turn of the century. London: Institute of Education.

Fine, M., & Weis, L. (1998). The unknown city: Lives of poor and working class young adults. Boston: Beacon Press.

Finkelhor, D. (1994). Current information on the scope and nature of child sexual abuse. The Future of Children, 4(2), 31–53.

Fish, M., Stifter, C. A., & Belsky, J. (1993). Early patterns of mother–infant dyadic interaction: Infant, mother, and family demographic antecedents. Infant Behavior & Development, 16(1), 1–18.

Flanagan, J. C., Cooley, W. W., Lohnes, P. R., Schoenfeldt, L. F., Holdeman, R. W., Combs, J., et al. (1966). Project TALENT one-year follow-up studies. Pittsburgh: American Institutes for Research.

Flanagan, J. C., Davis, F. B., Dailey, J. T., Shaycoft, M. F., Orr, D. B., Goldberg, I., et al. (1964). The American high school student: American Institutes for Research. Available online at: www.icpsr.umich.edu/cocoon/ICPSR/STUDY/07823.xml

Freedman, D. S., & Thornton, A. (1979). The long-term impact of pregnancy at marriage on the family's economic circumstances. Family Planning Perspectives, 11(1), 6–21.

Freese, J., Meland, S., & Irwin, W. (2007). Expressions of positive emotion in photographs, personality, and later-life marital and health outcomes. Journal of Research in Personality, 41(2), 488–497.

Friedman, H. S., Tucker, J. S., Schwartz, J. E., Tomlinson-Keasey, C., Martin, L. R., Wingard, D. L., et al. (1995). Psychosocial and behavioral predictors of longevity: The aging and death of the "termites." American Psychologist, 50 (2), 69–78.

Froehlich, G. J. (1941). The prediction of academic success at the University of Wisconsin, 1909–1941. Madison: Bureaus of Guidance and Records, University of Wisconsin.

Furstenberg, F. F., Jr., Cook, T. D., Eccles, J., Elder, G. H., Jr., & Sameroff, A. (Eds.). (1999). Managing to make it: Urban families and adolescent success. Chicago: University of Chicago Press.

Gager, C. T., & Sanchez, L. (2003). Two as one?: Couples' perception of time spent together, marital quality, and the risk of divorce. Journal of Family Issues, 24(1), 21–50.

Gale, J. (1992). When research interviews are more therapeutic than therapy interviews. The Qualitative Report, 1(4), 31–38.

Gans, H. J. (1968). The participant–observer as a human being: Observations on the personal aspects of fieldwork. In H. S. Becker, B. Geer, D. Riesman, & R. S. Weiss (Eds.), Institutions and the person (pp. 300–374). Chicago: Aldine.

Ge, X., Conger, R. D., Cadoret, R. J., Neiderhiser, J. M., Yates, W. R., Troughton, E., et al. (1996). The developmental interface between nature and nurture: A mutual influence model of child antisocial behavior and parent behaviors. Developmental Psychology, 32 (4), 574–589.

George, L. K. (1993). Sociological perspectives on life transitions. Annual Review of Sociology, 19, 353–373.

George, L. K., Larson, D. B., Koenig, H. G., & McCullough, M. (2000). Spirituality and health: State of the evidence. Journal of Social and Clinical Psychology, 19, 102–116.

George, L. K., & Lynch, S. M. (2003). Race differences in depressive symptoms: A dynamic perspective on stress exposure and vulnerability. Journal of Health and Social Behavior, 44(3), 353–369.

Geronimus, A. T. (1996). Black/white differences in the relationship of maternal age to birthweight: A population-based test of the weathering hypothesis. Social Science and Medicine, 42 (4), 589–597.

Gerstel, N. (2000). The third shift: Gender and care work outside the home. Qualitative Sociology, 23(4), 467–483.

Giarrusso, R., Feng, D., Silverstein, M., & Bengston, V. L. (2001). Grandparent—adult grandchild affection and consensus: Cross-generational and crossethnic comparisons. Journal of Family Issues, 22 (4), 456–477.

Giele, J. Z. (1987). Coeducation or women's education?: A comparison of findings from two colleges. In C. Lasser (Ed.), Coeducation: Past, present, and future (pp. 91–109). Urbana: University of Illinois Press.

Giele, J. Z. (1995). Two paths to women's equality: Temperance, suffrage, and the origins of modern feminism. New York: Twayne.

Giele, J. Z. (1998). Innovation in the typical life course. In J. Z. Giele & G. H. Elder, Jr. (Eds.), Methods of life course research: Qualitative and quantitative approaches (pp. 231–263). Thousand Oaks, CA: Sage.

Giele, J. Z. (2002a). Life course studies and the theory of action. In R. A. Settersten, Jr. & T. J. Owens (Eds.), Advances in life-course research: New frontiers in socialization (Vol. 7, pp. 65–88). London: Elsevier Science.

Giele, J. Z. (2002b). Longitudinal studies and life-course research: Innovations, investigators, and policy ideas. In E. Phelps, F. F. Furstenberg, Jr., & A. Colby (Eds.), Looking at lives: American longitudinal studies of the twentieth century (pp. 15–36). New York: Russell Sage Foundation.

Giele, J. Z. (2004). Women and men as agents of change in their own lives. In J. Z. Giele & E. Holst (Eds.), Advances in life course research: Changing life patterns in Western industrial societies (Vol. 8, pp. 299–317). Amsterdam: Elsevier Science.

Giele, J. Z. (2008). Homemaker or career woman: Life-course factors and racial influences in the American middle class. Journal of Comparative Family Studies, 39 (3), 392–411.

Giele, J. Z., & Elder, G. H., Jr. (1998a). Life course research: Development of a field. In Methods of life course research: Quantitative and qualitative approaches (pp. 5–27). Thousand Oaks, CA: Sage.

Giele, J. Z., & Elder, G. H., Jr. (Eds.). (1998b). Methods of life course research: Qualitative and quantitative approaches. Thousand Oaks, CA: Sage.

Giele, J. Z., & Gilfus, M. (1990). Race and college differences in life patterns of educated women. In J. Antler & S. Biklen (Eds.), Women and educational change (pp. 179–197). Albany: State University of New York Press.

Gill, T. M., Allore, H. G., Hardy, S. E., & Guo, Z. C. (2006). The dynamic nature of mobility disability in older persons. Journal of the American Geriatrics Society, 54(2), 248–254.

Glenn, N. (1977). Cohort analysis. Beverly Hills, CA: Sage.

Glueck, S., & Glueck, E. (1950). Unraveling juvenile delinquency. New York: New York Commonwealth Fund.

Glueck, S., & Glueck, E. (1968). Delinquents and nondelinquents in perspective. Cambridge, MA: Harvard University Press.

Goffman, E. (1959). The presentation of self in everyday life. Garden City, N Y: Doubleday.

Goffman, E. (1963). Stigma: Notes on the preservaton of spoiled identity. Englewood Cliffs, NJ: Prentice-Hall.

Gold, R. L. (1958). Roles in sociological field observations. Social Forces, 36(3), 217–223.

Gottfredson, M. R., & Hirschi, T. (1986). The true value of lambda would appear to be zero: An essay on career criminals, criminal careers, selective incapacitation, cohort studies, and related topics. Criminology, 24(2), 213–234.

Gottlieb, G. (2003). On making behavioral genetics truly developmental. Human Development, 46(6), 337–355.

Gottman, J.M., & Notarius, C.I. (2000). Decade review: Observing marital interaction. Journal of Marriage and the Family, 62 (4), 927–947.

Griffin, M.A., Patterson, M.G., & West, M.A. (2001). Job satisfaction and teamwork: The role of supervisor support. Journal of Organizational Behavior, 22 (5), 537–550.

Griffith, J. (2002). Multilevel analysis of cohesion's relation to stress, well-being, identification, disintegration, and perceived combat readiness. Military Psychology, 14(3), 217–239.

Guerrero, T.J., & Naldini, M. (1996). Is the South so different?: Italian and Spanish families in comparative perspective. In M. Rhodes (Ed.), Southern European welfare states: Between crisis and reform (Vol. 1, pp. 42–66). London: Frank Cass.

Guo, G., & Zhao, H. (2000). Multilevel modeling for binary data. Annual Review of Sociology, 26(1), 441–462.

Gurin, G., Veroff, J., & Feld, S. (1960). Americans view their mental health: A nationwide interview survey: A report to the staff director, Jack E. Ewalt. New York: Basic Books.

Guthrie, G.J., & Jenkins, S. (2005). Bertillon Files: An untapped source of nineteenth-century human height data. Journal of Anthropological Research, 61(2), 201–215.

Guttmann, M.P., & Fliess, K.H. (1993). The determinants of early fertility decline in Texas. Demography, 30 (3), 443–457.

Haas, S. (2008). Trajectories of functional health: The "long arm" of childhood health and socioeconomic factors. Social Science and Medicine, 66(4), 849–861.

Hall, C.S., & Lindzey, G. (1957). Theories of personality. New York: Wiley.

Hallqvist, J., Lynch, J., Bartley, M., Lang, T., & Blane, D. (2004). Can we disentangle life course processes of accumulation, critical period, and social mobility?: An analysis of disadvantaged socio-economic positions and myocardial infarction in the Stockholm Health Epidemiology Program. Social Science and Medicine, 58 (8), 1555–1562.

Hamil-Luker, J. (2005). Trajectories of public assistance receipt among female high school dropouts. Population Research and Policy Review, 24(6), 673–694.

Hamil-Luker, J., & O'Rand, A.M. (2007). Gender differences in the impact of childhood adversity on the risk for heart attack across the life course. Demography, 44(1), 137–158.

Hammack, P.L. (2008). Narrative and cultural psychology of identity. Personality and Social Psychology Review, 12 (3), 222–247.

Han, S.-K., & Moen, P. (1999). Clocking out: Temporal patterning of retirement. American Journal of Sociology, 105(1), 191–236.

Han, S.-K., & Moen, P. (2001). Coupled careers: Pathways through work and marriage in the United States. In H.-P. Blossfeld & S. Drobnic (Eds.), Careers of couples in contemporary societies: From male breadwinner to dual earner families (pp. 201–232). Oxford, England: Oxford University Press.

Hareven, T.K. (1978). Transitions: The family and the life course in historical perspective. New York: Academic Press.

Hareven, T.K. (1982). Family time and industrial time. New York: Cambridge University Press.

Harrington, B. (2003). The social psychology of access in ethnographic research. Journal of Contemporary Ethnography, 32(5), 592–625.

Hauser, R.M. (1984). Some cross-population comparisons of family bias in the effects of schooling on occupational status. Social Science Research, 13(2), 159–187.

Hauser, R. M. (1988). A note on two models of sibling resemblance. American Journal of Sociology, 93(6), 1401–1423.

Hauser, R. M. (2005). Survey response in the long run: The Wisconsin Longitudinal Study. Field Methods, 17, 3–29.

Hauser, R. M., & Dickinson, P. J. (1974). Inequality on occupational status and income. American Educational Research Journal, 11, 161–168.

Hauser, R. M., & Featherman, D. L. (1977). The process of stratification: Trends and analyses. New York: Academic Press.

Hauser, R. M., & Mossel, P. A. (1985). Fraternal resemblance in educational attainment and occupational status. American Journal of Sociology, 91(3), 650–673.

Hauser, R. M., & Mossel, P. A. (1988). Some structural equation models of sib ling resemblance in educational attainment and occupational status. In P. Cuttance & R. Ecob (Eds.), Structural modeling by example: Applications in educational, sociological, and behavioral research (pp. 108–137). Cambridge, England: Cambridge University Press.

Hauser, R. M., & Sewell, W. H. (1986). Family effects in simple models of education, occupational status, and earnings: Findings from the Wisconsin and Kalamazoo Studies. Journal of Labor Economics, 4(3, Part 2), S83–S115.

Hauser, R. M., Sheridan, J. T., & Warren, J. R. (1999). Socioeconomic achievements of siblings in the life course: New findings from the Wisconsin Longitudinal Study. Research on Aging, 21(2), 338–378.

Hauser, R. M., Tsai, S. L., & Sewell, W. H. (1983). A model of stratification with response error in social and psychological variables. Sociology of Education, 56(1), 20–46.

Hauser, R. M., Warren, J. R., Huang, M.-H., & Carter, W. Y. (2000). Occupational status, education, and social mobility in the meritocracy. In K. Arrow, S. Bowles, & S. Durlauf (Eds.), Meritocracy and economic inequality (pp. 179–229). Princeton, NJ: Princeton University Press.

Hauser, R. M., & Wong, R. S.-K. (1989). Sibling resemblance and inter-sibling effects in educational attainment. Sociology of Education, 62 (3), 149–171.

Hayward, M. D., & Gorman, B. K. (2004). The long arm of childhood: The influence of early-life social conditions on men's mortality. Demography, 41(1), 87–107.

Heckhausen, J. (1999). Developmental regulation in adulthood: Age-normative and sociostructural constraints as adaptive challenges. New York: Cambridge University Press.

Heinz, W. R. (1996). Status passages as micro–macro linkages in life course research. In A. Weymann & W. R. Heinz (Eds.), Society and biography: Interrelationships between social structure, institutions and the life course (pp. 67–81). Weinheim, Germany: Deutscher Studien Verlag.

Heinz, W. R. (2002). Transition discontinuities and the biographical shaping of early work careers. Journal of Vocational Behavior, 60 (2), 220–240.

Heise, D. R. (1990). Careers, career trajectories, and the self. In J. Rodin, C. Schooler, & K. W. Schaie (Eds.), Self-directedness: Cause and effects throughout the life course (pp. 59–84). Hillsdale, NJ: Erlbaum.

Henmon, V. A. C., & Holt, F. O. (1931). A report on the administration of scholastic aptitude tests to 34,000 high school seniors in Wisconsin in 1929 and 1930 prepared for the Committee on Cooperation, Wisconsin secondary schools and colleges. Madison: Bureau of Guidance and Records, University of Wisconsin.

Henmon, V. A. C., & Nelson, M. J. (1946). Henmon–Nelson Tests of Mental Ability, High School Examination—Grades 7 to 12—Forms A, B, and C: Teacher's manual. Boston: Houghton-Mifflin.

Henmon, V. A. C., & Nelson, M. J. (1954). The Henmon–Nelson Tests of Mental Ability: Manual for administration. Boston: Houghton-Mifflin.

Henretta, J.C., & Campbell, R.T. (1976). Status attainment and status maintenance: A study of stratification in old age. American Sociological Review, 41(6),
981–992.

Henry, B., Moffitt, T. E., Caspi, A., Langley, J., & Silva, P. A. (1994). On the "remem-
brance of things past": A longitudinal evaluation of the retrospective method.
Psychological Assessment, 6(2), 92–101.

Herd, P., Goesling, B., & House, J.S. (2007). Socioeconomic position and health:
The differential effects of education versus income on the onset versus progression of health problems. Journal of Health and Social Behavior, 48 (3), 223–238.

Hetherington, E.M., & Baltes, P.B. (1988). Child psychology and life-span development. In E.M. Hetherington, R.M. Lerner, & M. Perlmutter (Eds.), Child development in life-span perspective (pp. 1–19). Hillsdale, NJ: Erlbaum.

Higginbotham, E. (2001). Too much to ask: Black women in the era of integration.
Chapel Hill: University of North Carolina Press.

Higuchi, S., Matsushita, S., Imazeki, H., K inoshita, T., Takagi, S., & Kono, H.
(1994). Aldehyde dehydrogenase genotypes in Japanese alcoholics. Lancet, 343,
741–742.

Hill, R., & Foote, N.N. (1970). Family development in three generations: A longitudinal study of changing family patterns of planning and achievement. Cambridge,
MA: Schenkman.

Hirschi, T., & Gottfredson, M.R. (1983). Age and the explanation of crime. American Journal of Sociology, 89 (2), 552–584.

Hochschild, A.R. (1989). The second shift: Working parents and the revolution at
home. New York: Penguin Books.

Hogan, D.P. (1981). Transitions and social change: The early lives of American men.
New York: Academic Press.

Hogan, D.P., & Goldscheider, F.K. (2003). Success and challenge in demographic
studies of the life course. In J.T. Mortimer & M.J. Shanahan (Eds.), Handbook
of the life course (pp. 681–691). New York: K luwer Academic/Plenum Press.

Hogan, D.P., & Park, J.M. (2000). Family factors and social support in the developmental outcomes of children who were very low birthweight at 32 to 38 months
of age. Seminars in Perinatology, 27(2), 433–459.

Holahan, C.K., & Sears, R.R. (1995). The gifted group in later maturity. Stanford,
CA: Stanford University Press.

Holmes, T.H., & Rahe, R.H. (1967). The social readjustment rating scale. Journal
of Psychosomatic Research, 11, 213–218.

House, J.S., Lantz, P.M., & Herd, P. (2005). Continuity and change in the social
stratification of aging and health over the life course: Evidence from a nationally
representative Longitudinal Study from 1986 to 2001/2 (Americans' Changing
Lives Study). Journals of Gerontology B: Psychological Sciences and Social Sciences, 60 (Special Issue 2), S15–S26.

Howe, M.J. (1982). Biographical evidence and the development of outstanding individuals. American Psychologist, 37(10), 1071–1081.

Hughes, D.C., Blazer, D.G., & George, L.K. (1988). Age differences in life events:
A multivariate controlled analysis. International Journal of Aging and Human
Development, 27(3), 207–220.

Huinink, J. (1989). Mehrebenenanalyse in den Sozialwissenschaften [Multi-level
analysis in the social sciences]. Wiesbaden: Deutscher Universitäs-Verlag.

Hultsch, D.F., & Plemons, J.K. (1979). Life events and life-span development. In
P.B. Baltes & O.G. Brim (Eds.), Life-span development and behavior (Vol. 2,
pp. 1–36). New York: Academic Press.

Human Capital Initiative Coordinating Committee on Reducing Violence. (1995).
Report presented at Reducing Violence: A Research Agenda, Washington, DC.

Hyman, H. H. (1972). Secondary analysis of sample surveys: Principles, procedures, and potentialities. New York: Wiley.

Hynes, K., & Clarkberg, M. (2005). Women's employment patterns during early parenthood: A group-based trajectory analysis. Journal of Marriage and the Family, 67(1), 222–239.

Jacobs, J. A., & Gerson, K. (2004). The time divide: Work, family, and gender inequality. Cambridge, MA: Harvard University Press.

Jaffee, S. R., & Price, T. S. (2007). Gene–environment correlations: A review of the evidence and implications for prevention of mental illness. Molecular Psychiatry, 12 (5), 432–442.

Jagger, C., Matthews, R., Melzer, D., Matthews, F., Brayne, C., & MRC-CFAS. (2007). Educational differences in the dynamics of disability incidence, recovery, and mortality: Findings from the MRC Cognitive Function and Ageing Study. International Journal of Epidemiology, 36(2), 358–365.

Janoski, T., & Hicks, A. M. E. (1994). The comparative political economy of the welfare state. Cambridge, England: Cambridge University Press.

Janson, C.-G. (1990). Retrospective data, undesirable behavior, and the longitudinal perspective. In D. Magnusson & L. R. Bergman (Eds.), Data quality in longitudinal research (pp. 100–121). Cambridge, England: Cambridge University Press.

Jarvie, I. C. (1969). The problem of ethical integrity in participant observation. Current Anthropology, 10 (5), 505–508.

Jencks, C., Smith, M., Acland, H., Bane, M. J., Cohen, D., Gintis, H., et al. (1972). Inequality: A reassessment of the effect of family and schooling in America. New York: Basic Books.

Johnson, M. K. (2002). Social origins, adolescent experiences, and work value trajectories during the transition to adulthood. Social Forces, 80 (4), 1307–1341.

Johnson, W. (2007). Genetic and environmental influences on behavior: Capturing all the interplay. Psychological Review, 114(2), 423–440.

Johnson, W., & K rueger, R. F. (2004). Genetic and environmental structure of adjectives describing the domains of the Big Five model of personality: A nationwide U.S. twin study. Journal of Research on Personality, 38 (5), 448–472.

Jones, B. L., Nagin, D. S., & Roeder, K. (2001). A SAS procedure based on mixture models for estimating developmental trajectories. Sociological Methods and Research, 29 (3), 374–393.

Jordan, N. C., Kaplan, D., Olah, L. N., & Locuniak, M. N. (2006). Number sense growth in kindergarten: A longitudinal investigation of children at risk for mathematical difficulties. Child Development, 77(1), 153–175.

Jöreskog, K. G., & Sörbom, D. (1996). LISR EL 8 user's reference guide. Chicago: Scientific Software International.

Jouriles, E. N., McDonald, R., Norwood, W. D., & Ezell, E. (2001). Issues and controversies in documenting the prevalence of children's exposure to domestic violence. In S. A. Graham-Bermann & J. L. Edleson (Eds.), Domestic violence in the lives of children: The future of research, intervention, and social policy (pp. 12–34). Washington, DC : American Psychological Association.

Kahn, R. L., & Antonucci, T. C. (1980). Convoys over the life course: Attachment, roles, and social support. In P. B. Baltes & O. G. Brim, Jr. (Eds.), Lifespan development and behavior (Vol. 3, pp. 253–286). New York: Academic Press.

Karweit, N., & Kertzer, D. I. (1998). Data organization and conceptualization. In J. Z. Giele & G. H. Elder, Jr. (Eds.), Methods of life course research: Qualitative and quantitative approaches (pp. 81–97). Thousand Oaks, CA: Sage.

Kelley-Moore, J. A., & Ferraro, K. F. (2004). The black/white disability gap: Persistent inequality in later life? Journal of Gerontology B: Psychological Sciences and Social Sciences, 59 (1), S34–S43.

Kendler, K. S., Neale, M., Kessler, R. C., Heath, A. C., & Eaves, L. (1993). A longitudinal twin study of personality and major depression in women. Archives of General Psychiatry, 50 (11), 853–862.

Kendler, K. S., Thornton, L. M., & Pedersen, N. L. (2000). Tobacco consumption in Swedish twins reared apart and reared together. Archives of General Psychiatry, 87(9), 886–892.

Kerckhoff, A. C. (1976). The status attainment process: Socialization or allocation? Social Forces, 55, 368–381.

Kerckhoff, A. C. (1989). On the social psychology of social mobility processes. Social Forces, 68 (1), 17–25.

Kertzer, D. I., & Hogan, D. P. (1989). Family, political economy, and demographic change: The transformation of life in Casalecchio, Italy, 1861–1921. Madison: University of Wisconsin Press.

Kessler, R. C., & Greenberg, D. F. (1981). Linear panel analysis: Models of quantitative change. New York: Academic Press.

Kidwell, R. E., Jr., Mossholder, K. W., & Bennett, N. (1997). Cohesiveness and organizational citizenship behavior: A multilevel analysis using work groups and individuals. Journal of Management, 23(6), 775–793.

Kiecolt-Glaser, J. K., & Newton, T. L. (2001). Marriage and health: His and hers. Psychological Bulletin, 127(4), 472–503.

Kim-Cohen, J., Caspi, A., Taylor, A., Williams, B., Newcombe, R., Craig, I. W., et al. (2006). MAOA, maltreatment, and gene–environment interaction predicting children's mental health: New evidence and a meta-analysis. Molecular Psychiatry, 11(10), 903–913.

Kirchler, E., Rodler, C., Holzl, E., & Meier, K. (2001). Conflict and decision-making in close relationships: Love, money and daily routines. East Sussex, England: Psychology Press.

Kleinman, S. (1991). Field-workers' feelings: What we feel, who we are, how we analyze. In W. B. Shaffir & R. A. Stebbins (Eds.), Experiencing fieldwork: An inside view of qualitative research (pp. 184–195). Newbury Park, CA: Sage.

Kleinman, S., & Copp, M. A. (1993). Emotions and fieldwork. Newbury Park, CA: Sage.

Kloos, P. (1969). Role conflicts in social fieldwork. Current Anthropology, 10 (5), 509–512.

Knaub, P. K., Eversoll, D. B., & Voss, J. H. (1983). Is parenthood a desirable adult role?: An assessment of attitudes held by contemporary women. Sex Roles, 9 (3), 355–362.

Kohli, M. (1981). Biography: Account, text, method. In D. Bertaux (Ed.), Biography and society: The life history approach in the social sciences (pp. 61–75). Beverly Hills, CA: Sage.

Kohn, M. L. (1987). Cross-national research as an analytic strategy. American Sociological Review, 52 (6), 713–731.

Kohn, M. L., & Schooler, C. (1983). Work and personality: An inquiry into the impact of social stratification. Norwood, NJ: Ablex.

Komarovsky, M. (1985). Women in college: Shaping new feminine identities. New York: Basic Books.

Komlos, J. (2004). How to (and how not to) analyze deficient height samples. Historical Methods, 37(4), 160–173.

Kreuter, F., & Muthén, B. (2008). Analyzing criminal trajectory profiles: Bridging multilevel and group-based approaches using growth mixture modeling. Journal of Quantitative Criminology, 24(1), 1–31.

Kuh, D., & Ben-Shlomo, Y. (2004). A life course approach to chronic disease epidemiology. New York: Oxford University Press. (Original work published 1997)

Kurtines, W. M., Ferrer-Wreder, L., Berman, S. L., Lorente, C. C., Briones, E., Montgomery, M. J., et al. (2008). Promoting positive youth development: The Miami Youth Development Project (Y DP). Journal of Adolescent Research, 23(3), 256–267.

Kurz, D. (1996). Separation, divorce, and woman abuse. Violence Against Women, 2(1), 63–81.

Lachman, M. E., & Weaver, S. L. (1998). Sociodemographic variations in the sense of control by domain: Findings from the MacArthur studies on midlife. Psychology and Aging, 13(4), 553–562.

Land, K. C., McCall, P. L., & Nagin, D. S. (1996). A comparison of Poisson, negative binomial, and semiparametric mixed Poisson regression models with empirical applications to criminal careers data. Sociological Methods and Research, 24(4), 387–442.

Larson, R. W., & Almeida, D. M. (1999). Emotional transmission in the daily lives of families: A new paradigm for studying family process. Journal of Marriage and the Family, 61(1), 5–20.

Laub, J. H. (2006). Edwin H. Sutherland and the Michael–Adler report: Searching for the soul of criminology 70 years later: The 2005 Sutherland Award address. Criminology, 44(2), 235–258.

Laub, J. H., Nagin, D., & Sampson, R. J. (1998). Trajectories of change in criminal offending: Good marriages and the desistance process. American Sociological Review, 63, 225–238.

Laub, J. H., & Sampson, R. J. (1993). Turning points in the life course: Why change matters to the study of crime. Criminology, 31(3), 301–325.

Laub, J. H., & Sampson, R. J. (2002). Sheldon and Eleanor Gluecks' Unraveling Juvenile Delinquency Study: The lives of 1,000 Boston men in the twentieth century. In E. Phelps, F. F. Furstenberg, Jr., & A. Colby (Eds.), Looking at lives: American longitudinal studies of the twentieth century (pp. 87–115). New York: Russell Sage Foundation.

Laub, J. H., & Sampson, R. J. (2003). Shared beginnings, divergent lives. Cambridge, MA: Harvard University Press.

Lauderdale, D. S., & Kestenbaum, B. (2002). Mortality rates of elderly Asian American populations based on Medicare and Social Security data. Demography, 36(3), 529–540.

Lazarfield, P. F., Berelson, B., & Gaudet, H. (1994). The people's choice: How the voter makes up his mind in a presidential campaign (Columbia University Bureau of Applied Research No. B-3). New York: Duell, Sloane, & Pierce. Lazarus, R. S. (1996). The role of coping in the emotions and how coping changes over the life course. In C. Malatesta-Magai & S. H. McFadden (Eds.), Handbook of emotion, adult development and aging (pp. 289–306). New York: Academic Press.

Lazarus, R. S. (1999). Stress and emotion: A new synthesis. New York: Springer.

Leone, J. M., Johnson, M. P., Cohan, C. L., & Lloyd, S. E. (2004). Consequences of male partner violence for low-income minority women. Journal of Marriage and Family, 66(2), 472–490.

Lieberson, S. (1985). Making it count: The improvement of social research and theory. Berkeley: University of California Press.

Link, B. G., & Phelan, J. (1995). Social conditions as fundamental causes of disease. Journal of Health and Social Behavior, 35(Extra issue: Forty Years of Medical Sociology: The State of the Art and Directions for the Future), 80–94.

Little, J. K. (1958). A state-wide inquiry into decisions of youth about education beyond high school—follow-up studies. Madison: University of Wisconsin School of Education.

Little, J. K. (1959). Explorations into the college plans and experiences of high school graduates: A state-wide inquiry. Madison: University of Wisconsin School of Education.

Loeber, R., & Hay, D. (1997). Key issues in the development of aggression and violence from childhood to early adulthood. Annual Review of Psychology, 48 (1), 371–410.

Lorenz, F. O., Wickrama, K. A. S., Conger, R. D., & Elder, G. H., Jr. (2006). The short-term and decade-long effects of divorce on women's midlife health. Journal of Health and Social Behavior, 47(2), 111–125.

Lowenthal, M. F., & Chiriboga, D. A. (1972). Transition to the empty nest: Crisis, change, or relief ? Archives of General Psychiatry, 26(1), 8–14.

Lowenthal, M. F., Thurnher, M., & Chiriboga, D. A. (1975). Four stages of life: A comparative study of men and women facing transitions. San Francisco: JosseyBass.

Lunney, J. R., Lynn, J., Foley, D. J., Lipson, S., & Guralnik, J. M. (2003). Patterns of functional decline at the end of life. Journal of the American Medical Association, 289 (18), 2387–2392.

Luo, Y., & Waite, L. J. (2005). The impact of childhood and adult SES on physical, mental, and cognitive well-being in later life. Journals of Gerontology B: Psychological Sciences and Social Sciences, 60 (2), 93–101.

Luster, T., Small, S. A., & Lower, R. (2002). The correlates of abuse and witnessing abuse among adolescents. Journal of Interpersonal Violence, 17(12), 1323–1340.

Lynch, S. M. (2003). Cohort and life-course patterns in the relationship between education and health: A hierarchical approach. Demography, 40 (2), 309–331.

Lynch, S. M., & George, L. K. (2002). Interlocking trajectories of loss-related events and depressive symptoms among elders. Journals of Gerontology B: Psychological Sciences and Social Sciences, 57(2), S117–S125.

Lynn, J. (1997). An 88-year-old woman facing the end of life. Journal of the American Medical Association, 277(20), 925–932.

Lynn, J. (2001). Serving patients who may die soon and their families: The role of hospice and other services. Journal of the American Medical Association, 285(7), 925–932.

Macmillan, R. (2001). Violence and the life course: The consequences of victimization for personal and social development. Annual Review of Sociology, 27, 1–22.

Magnusson, D. (1988). Individual development from an interactional perspective: A longitudinal study. Hillsdale, NJ: Erlbaum.

Maguire, M. C. (1999). Treating the dyad as the unit of analysis: A primer on three analytic approaches. Journal of Marriage and the Family, 61(1), 213–223.

Manting, D. (1996). The changing meaning of cohabitation and marriage. European Sociological Review, 12 (1), 53–65.

Marmot, M. G., Smith, G. D., Stansfeld, S., Patel, C., North, F., Head, J., et al. (1991). Health inequalities among British civil servants: The Whitehall II study. Lancet, 337(8754), 1387–1393.

Martijn, C., & Sharpe, L. (2006). Pathways to youth homelessness. Social Science and Medicine, 62 (1), 1–12.

Mason, C. M., & Griffin, M. A. (2003). Group absenteeism and positive affective tone: A longitudinal study. Journal of Organizational Behavior, 24(6), 667–687.

Mason, W. M., & Fienberg, S. E. E. (1985). Cohort analysis in social research. New York: Springer.

Mayer, K. U. (1990). Lebensverläufe und sozialer Wandel. Sonderheft 31, Kölner Zeitschrift für Soziologie und Sozialpsychologie [Life courses and social change. Kölner Journal of Sociology and Social Psychology.] Special edition 31. Opladen: Westdeutscher Verlag.

Mayer, K. U. (1997). Notes on a comparative political economy of life courses. Comparative Social Research, 16, 203–226.

Mayer, K. U. (2009). New directions in life course research. Annual Review of Sociology, 35, 20.1–20.21.

Mayer, K. U., & Huinink, J. (1990). Age, period, and cohort in the study of the life course: A comparison of classical A-P-C analysis with event history analysis or farewell to Lexis? In D. Magnusson & L. R. Bergman (Eds.), Data quality in longitudinal research (pp. 211–232). New York: Cambridge University Press.

Mayer, K. U., & Tuma, N. B. (Eds.). (1990). Event history analysis in life course research. Madison: University of Wisconsin Press.

McAdams, D. P. (1985). Power, intimacy, and the life story: Personological inquiries into identity. Homewood, IL: Dorsey Press.

McAdam, D. (1989). The biographical consequences of activism. American Sociological Review, 54, 744–760.

McAdams, D. P. (2001). The psychology of life stories. Review of General Psychology, 5(2), 100–122.

McAdams, D. P. (2006). The redemptive self: Generativity and the stories Americans live by. Research in Human Development, 3(2 & 3), 81–100.

McClelland, D.C. (1967). The achieving society. New York: Free Press. McClelland, D.C. (1975). Power: The inner experience. New York: Irvington. McDonough, P., & Berglund, P. (2003). Histories of poverty and self-rated health trajectories. Journal of Health and Social Behavior, 44(2), 198–214. McGue, M., & Christensen, K. (2003). The heritability of depression symptoms in elderly Danish twins: Occasion-specific versus general effects. Behavior Genetics, 33(2), 83–93.

McLeod, J. D., & Almazan, E. P. (2003). Connections between childhood and adulthood. In J. T. Mortimer & M. J. Shanahan (Eds.), Handbook of the life course (pp. 391–412). New York: K luwer Academic/Plenum Press.

McLeod, J. D., & Fettes, D. L. (2007). Trajectories of failure: The educational careers of children with mental health problems. American Journal of Sociology, 113(3), 653–701.

Mead, M. (1963). Sex and temperament in three primitive societies. New York: Morrow.

Meland, S. A. (2002). Objectivity in perceived attractiveness: Development of a new methodology for rating facial physical attractiveness. Unpublished MA thesis, Department of Sociology, University of Wisconsin–Madison.

Menard, S. (Ed.). (2008). Handbook of longitudinal research: Design, measurement, and analysis. Burlington, MA: Elsevier.

Merton, R. K. (1957). Puritanism, pietism, and science. In Social theory and social structure (pp. 574–606). Glencoe, IL: Free Press. (Original work published 1949)

Merton, R. K. (1959). Notes on problem finding in sociology. In R. K. Merton, L. Broom, & L. S. Cottrell, Jr. (Eds.), Sociology today: Problems and prospects (pp. ix–xxxiv). New York: Basic Books.

Merton, R. K. (1968). The Matthew effect in science. Science, 159 (3810), 56–63.

Miles, M. B., & Huberman, A. M. (1994). Qualitative data analysis: An expanded sourcebook (2nd ed.). Thousand Oaks, CA: Sage.

Minton, H. L. (1988a). Charting life history: Lewis M. Terman's study of the gifted. In J. G. Morawski (Ed.), The rise of experimentation in American psychology (pp. 138–162). New Haven, CT: Yale University Press.

Minton, H. L. (1988b). Lewis M. Terman: Pioneer in psychological testing. New York: New York University Press.

Mirowsky, J., & Ross, C. E. (2003). Education, social status, and health. New York: de Gruyter.

Mishler, E. G. (1996). Missing persons: Recovering developmental stories/histories. In R. Jessor, A. Colby, & R. A. Schweder (Eds.), Ethnography and human development: Context and meaning in social inquiry (pp. 73–99). Chicago: University of Chicago Press.

Modell, J. (1989). Into one's own: From youth to adulthood in the United States 1920–1975. Berkeley: University of California Press.

Moen, P. (2003). Midcourse: Navigating retirement and a new life stage. In J. T. Mortimer & M. J. Shanahan (Eds.), Handbook of the life course (pp. 269–291). New York: K luwer Academic/Plenum Press.

Moen, P., & Chesley, N. (2008). Toxic job ecologies, time convoys, and work–family conflict: Can families (re)gain control and life course "fit"? In K. Korabik, D. S. Lero, & D. L. Whitehead (Eds.), Handbook of work–family integration: Research, theory, and best practices (pp. 95–122). New York: Elsevier.

Moen, P., Dempster-McClain, D., & Williams, R. M., Jr. (1989). Social integration and longevity: An event history analysis of women's roles and resilience. American Sociological Review, 54, 635–647.

Moen, P., Dempster-McClain, D., & Williams, R. M., Jr. (1992). Successful aging: A life-course perspective on women's multiple roles and health. American Journal of Sociology, 97(6), 1612–1638.

Moen, P., Erickson, M. A., & Dempster-McClain, D. (1997). Their mothers' daughters?: The intergenerational transmission of gender role orientations in a world of changing roles. Journal of Marriage and the Family, 59 (2), 281–293.

Moen, P., & Orrange, R. M. (2002). Careers and lives: Socialization, structural lag, and gendered ambivalence. In R. A. Settersten, Jr. & T. J. Owens (Eds.), Advances in life course research: New frontiers in socialization (Vol. 7, pp. 231–260). London: Elsevier Science.

Moen, P., & Roehling, P. (2005). The career mystique: Cracks in the American dream. Boulder, CO: Rowman & Littlefield.

Moen, P., & Sweet, S. (2002). Two careers, one employer: Couples working for the same corporation. Journal of Vocational Behavior, 61(3), 466–483.

Moen, P., & Sweet, S. (2003). Time clocks: Work-hour strategies. In P. Moen (Ed.), It's about time: Couples and careers (pp. 17–34). Ithaca, N Y: Cornell University Press.

Moen, P., Sweet, S., & Swisher, R. (2005). Embedded career clocks: The case of retirement planning. In R. Macmillan (Ed.), Advances in life course research: The structure of the life course: Individualized? Standardized? Differentiated? (Vol. 9, pp. 237–265). New York: Elsevier.

Moffitt, T. E. (1993). Adolescence-limited and life-course-persistent antisocial behavior: A developmental taxonomy. Psychological Review, 100 (4), 674–701.

Moffitt, T. E., Caspi, A., Harrington, H., & Milne, B. J. (2002). Males on the lifecourse-persistent and adolescence-limited antisocial pathways: Follow-up at age 26 years. Development and Psychopathology, 14(1), 179–207.

Moffitt, T. E., Caspi, A., & Rutter, M. (2005). Strategy for investigating interactions between measured genes and measured environments. Archives of General Psychiatry, 62 (5), 473–481.

Morrison, D. R., & Ritualo, A. (2000). Routes to children's economy recovery after divorce: Are cohabitation and remarriage equivalent? American Sociological Review, 65(4), 560–580.

Mortimer, J. T. (2003). Working and growing up in America. Cambridge, MA: Harvard University Press.

Mortimer, J. T., & Shanahan, M. J. (Eds.). (2003). Handbook on the life course. New York: K luwer Academic/Plenum Press.

Mroczek, D. K., & Kolarz, C. M. (1998). The effect of age on positive and negative affect: A developmental perspective on happiness. Journal of Personality and Social Psychology, 75(5), 1333–1349.

Murray, H. A. (1938). Explorations in personality: A clinical and experimental study of fifty men of college age. New York: Oxford University Press.

Murray, S. A., Kendall, M., Boyd, K., & Sheikh, A. (2005). Illness trajectories and palliative care. British Medical Journal, 330 (7498), 1007–1008.

Musick, J. S. (1993). Young, poor, and pregnant: The psychology of teenage motherhood. New Haven, CT: Yale University Press.

Musick, M. A., House, J. S., & Williams, D. R. (2004). Attendance at religious services and mortality in a national sample. Journal of Health and Social Behavior, 45(2), 198–213.

Mustillo, S., Worthman, C., Erkanli, A., Keeler, G., Angold, A., & Costello, E. J. (2003). Obesity and psychiatric disorder: Developmental trajectories. Pediatrics, 111(4), 851–859.

Muthén, B. (2001). Latent variable mixture modeling. In G. A. Marcoulides & R. E. Schumacker (Eds.), New developments and techniques in structural equation modeling (pp. 1–33). Mahwah, NJ: Erlbaum.

Muthén, B. (2004). Latent variable analysis: Growth mixtures modeling and related techniques for longitudinal data. In D. W. Kaplan (Ed.), Handbook of quantitative methodology for the social sciences (pp. 345–368). Newbury Park, CA: Sage.

Muthén, B., & Muthén, L. K. (2000). Integrating person-centered and variablecentered analysis: Growth mixture modeling with latent trajectory classes. Alcoholism: Clinical and Experimental Research, 24(6), 882–891.

Nagin, D. S. (1999). Analyzing developmental trajectories: A semiparametric group-based approach. Psychological Methods, 4(2), 139–157.

Nagin, D. S. (2005). Group-based modeling of development over the life course. Cambridge, MA: Harvard University Press.

Nagin, D. S., Farrington, D. P., & Moffitt, T. E. (1995). Life-course trajectories of different types of offenders. Criminology, 33(1), 111–139.

Nagin, D. S., & Land, K. C. (1993). Age, criminal careers and population heterogeneity: Specification and estimation of a nonparametric, mixed poisson model. Criminology, 31, 327–362.

Nagin, D. S., & Tremblay, R. E. (1999). Trajectories of boys' physical aggression, opposition, and hyperactivity on the path to physically violent and nonviolent juvenile delinquency. Child Development, 70 (5), 1181–1196.

Nagin, D., & Tremblay, R. E. (2005a). What has been learned from group-based trajectory modeling?: Examples from physical aggression and other problem behaviors. Annals of the American Academy of Political and Social Science, 602, 82–117.

Nagin, D. S., & Tremblay, R. E. (2005b). Developmental trajectory groups: Fact or a useful statistical fiction? Criminology, 43(4), 873–904.

Nansel, T. R., Haynie, D. L., & Simons-Morton, B. G. (2003). The association of bullying and victimization with middle school adjustment. In M. J. Elias & J. E. Zins (Eds.), Bullying, peer harassment, and victimization in the schools: The next generation of prevention (pp. 45–61). New York: Hawthorn Press.

National Center for Health Statistics. (1994). National Death Index: General description. Hyattsville, MD: U.S. Department of Health and Human Services, Public Health Service, Centers for Disease Control and Prevention, National Center for Health Statistics.

National Center for Health Statistics. (1999). NDI PLUS: Coded causes of death (rev. July 23, 1999 ed.). Hyattsville, MD: Division of Vital Statistics, National Center for Health Statistics, Centers for Disease Control and Prevention.

National Research Council. (2000). The aging mind: Opportunities in cognitive research. Washington, DC : National Academies Press.

National Research Council. (2001). Cells and surveys: Should biological measures be included in social science research? Washington, DC : National Academies Press.

National Research Council. (2006a). Genes, behavior, and the social environment: Moving beyond the nature/nurture debate. Washington, DC : National Academies Press.

National Research Council. (2006b). When I'm 64. Washington, DC : National Academies Press.

National Research Council. (2008). Biosocial surveys. Washington, DC : National Academies Press.

Nazio, T., & Blossfeld, H.-P. (2003). The diffusion of cohabitation among young women in West Germany, East Germany and Italy. European Journal of Population, 19 (1), 47–82.

Nesselroade, J. R., & Baltes, P. B. (1974). Adolescent personality development and historical change: 1970–1972. Monographs of the Society for Research in Child Development, 39 (1, Serial No. 154), 1–80.

Neugarten, B. L. (1979). Time, age, and the life cycle. American Journal of Psychiatry, 136(7), 887–894.

Neugarten, B. L., with a foreword by Dail A. Neugarten. (1996). The meanings of age: Selected papers of Bernice L. Neugarten. Chicago: University of Chicago Press.

Neupert, S. D., Almeida, D. M., & Charles, S. T. (2007). Age differences in reactivity to daily stressors: The role of personal control. Journals of Gerontology B: Psychological Sciences and Social Sciences, 62 (4), 216–225.

Neupert, S. D., Almeida, D. M., Mroczek, D. K., & Spiro, A., III. (2006). The effects of the Columbia shuttle disaster on the daily lives of older adults: Findings from the VA Normative Aging Study. Aging and Mental Health, 10 (3), 272–281.

Newman, K. S., & Massengill, R. P. (2006). The texture of hardship: Qualitative sociology of poverty. Annual Review of Sociology, 32, 423–446.

Nisbet, R. A. (1969). Social change and history: Aspects of Western theory development. New York: Oxford University Press.

Northouse, L. L., Mood, D., Templin, T., Mellon, S., & George, T. (2000). Couples' patterns of adjustment to colon cancer. Social Science and Medicine, 50 (2), 271–284.

Oden, M. H. (1968). The fulfillment of promise: 40-year follow-up of the Terman Gifted Group. Genetic Psychology Monographs, 77(1), 3–93.

Ong, A., Bergeman, C. S., & Bisconti, T. L. (2005). Unique effects of daily perceived control on anxiety symptomatology during conjugal bereavement. Personality and Individual Differences, 38 (3), 1057–1067.

O'Rand, A. M. (1996). The precious and the precocious: Understanding cumulative dis/advantage over the life course. The Gerontologist, 36, 230–238.

O'Rand, A. M. (2002). Cumulative advantage theory in life course research. Annual Review of Gerontology and Geriatrics, 22, 14–20.

O'Rand, A. M., & Hamil-Luker, J. (2005). Processes of cumulative adversity: Childhood disadvantage and increased risk of heart attack across the life course. Journals of Gerontology B: Psychological Sciences and Social Sciences, 60 (Special Issue 2), 117–124.

Orbuch, T. L., Thornton, A., & Cancio, J. (2000). The impact of marital quality, divorce, and remarriage on the relationships between parents and their children. Marriage and Family Review, 29 (4), 221–246.

Orcutt, H. K., Erikson, D. J., & Wolfe, J. (2004). The course of PTSD symptoms among Gulf War veterans: A growth mixture modeling approach. Journal of Traumatic Stress, 17(3), 195–202.

Ortiz, S. M. (2004). Leaving the private world of wives of professional athletes: A male sociologist's reflections. Journal of Contemporary Ethnography, 33(4), 466–487.

Osgood, D. W. (2005). Making sense of crime and the life course. Annals of the American Academy of Political and Social Science, 602, 196–211.

Palloni, A. (2006). Reproducing inequalities: Luck, wallets and the enduring effects of childhood health. Demography, 43(4), 587–616.

Pampel, F. C., & Rogers, R. G. (2004). Socioeconomic status, smoking and health: A test of competing theories of cumulative advantage. Journal of Health and Social Behavior, 45(3), 306–321.

Park, J. M., Hogan, D. P., & Goldscheider, F. K. (2003). Child disability and mothers' tubal sterilization. Perspectives on Sexual and Reproductive Health, 35(3), 138–143.

Parsons, T. (1966). Societies: Evolutionary and comparative perspectives. Englewood Cliffs, NJ: Prentice-Hall.

Parsons, T., Bales, R. F., & Shils, E. A. (1953). Working papers in the theory of action. Glencoe, IL: Free Press.

Patterson, G. R., & Yoerger, K. (1993). Developmental models for delinquent behavior. In S. Hodgins (Ed.), Mental disorder and crime (pp. 140–172). Newbury Park, CA: Sage.

Pavalko, E. K., & Elder, G. H., Jr. (1993). Women behind the men: Variations in wives' support of husbands' careers. Gender and Society, 7(4), 548–567.

Pavalko, E. K., & Smith, B. (1999). The rhythm of work: Health effects of women's work dynamics. Social Forces, 77(3), 1141–1162.

Pavalko, E. K., & Woodbury, S. (2000). Social roles as process: Caregiving careers and women's health. Journal of Health and Social Behavior, 41(1), 91–105.

Pearlin, L. I. (1999). The stress process revisited: Reflections on concepts and their interrelationships. In C. S. Aneshensel & J. C. Phelan (Eds.), Handbook of the sociobiology of mental health (pp. 395–415). New York: Kluwer.

Pearlin, L. I., Menaghan, E. G., Lieberman, M. A., & Mullan, J. T. (1981). The stress process. Journal of Health and Social Behavior, 22, 337–356.

Pearlin, L. I., Schieman, S., Fazio, E. M., & Meersman, S. C. (2005). Stress, health, and the life course: Some conceptual perspectives. Journal of Health and Social Behavior, 46(2), 205–219.

Pearlin, L. I., & Schooler, C. (1978). The structure of coping. Journal of Health and Social Behavior, 19 (1), 2–21.

Pearlin, L. I., & Skaff, M. M. (1996). Stress and the life course: A paradigmatic alliance. Gerontologist, 36(2), 239–247.

Pearlman, L. A., & Saakvitne, K. W. (1995). Trauma and the therapist: Countertransference and vicarious traumatization in psychotherapy with incest survivors. New York: Norton.

Pedersen, N. L., & Reynolds, C. A. (1998). Stability and change in adult personality: Genetic and environmental components. European Journal of Personality, 12 (5), 365–386.

Pellegrini, A. D. (2002). Bullying and victimization in middle school: A dominance relations perspective. Educational Psychologist, 37(3), 151–163.

Peterson, C., Seligman, M. E. P., Yurko, K. H., Martin, L. R., & Friedman, H. S. (1998). Catastrophizing and untimely death. Psychological Science, 9 (2), 127–130.

Peterson, R. R. (1996). A re-evaluation of the economic consequences of divorce. American Sociological Review, 61(2), 528–536.

Pettigrew, T. F. (1998). Intergroup conflict theory. Annual Review of Psychology, 49, 65–85.

Phelan, J. C., Link, B. G., Diez-Roux, A., Kawachi, I., & Levin, B. (2004). "Fundamental causes" of social inequalities in mortality: A test of the theory. Journal of Health and Social Behavior, 45(3), 265–285.

Phelps, E., Furstenberg, F. F., Jr., & Colby, A. (Eds.). (2002). Looking at lives: American longitudinal studies of the twentieth century. New York: Russell Sage Foundation.

Piquero, A. R. (2008). Taking stock of developmental trajectories of criminal activity over the life course. In A. Liberman (Ed.), The long view of crime: A synthesis of longitudinal research (pp. 23–78). New York: Springer.

Pixley, J. E. (2008). Life course patterns of career-prioritizing decisions and occupational attainment in dual-earner couples. Work and Occupations, 35(2), 127–163.

Plomin, R., DeFries, J. C., & Loehlin, J. C. (1977). Genotype–environment interaction and correlation in the analysis of human behavior. Psychological Bulletin, 84(2), 309–322.

Plomin, R., Pedersen, N. L., Lichtenstein, P., & McClearn, G. E. (1994). Variability and stability in cognitive abilities are largely genetic later in life. Behavior Genetics, 24(3), 207–215.

Pollner, M., & Emerson, R. M. (1983). The dynamics of inclusion and distance in fieldwork relations. In R. M. Emerson (Ed.), Contemporary field research: A collection of readings (pp. 235–252). Boston: Little, Brown.

Porter, J. N. (1974). Race, socialization and occupational mobility in educational and early occupational attainment. American Sociological Review, 39 (3), 303–316.

Portes, A., & Wilson, K. (1976). Black–white differences in educational attainment. American Sociological Review, 41(3), 414–431.

Purvin, D. M. (2003). Weaving a tangled safety net—the intergenerational legacy of domestic violence and poverty. Violence Against Women, 9 (10), 1263–1277.

Purvin, D. M. (2007). At the crossroads and in the crosshairs: Social welfare policy and low-income women's vulnerability to domestic violence. Social Problems, 54(2), 188–210.

Quick, H. E., & Moen, P. (1998). Gender, employment, and retirement quality: A life course approach to the differential experiences of men and women. Journal of Occupational Health Psychology, 3(1), 44–64.

Ragin, C. C. (1987). The comparative method: Moving beyond qualitative and quantitative strategies. Berkeley: University of California Press.

Ragin, C. C. (2000). Fuzzy-set social science. Chicago: University of Chicago Press.

Raley, S. B., Mattingly, M. J., & Bianchi, S. M. (2006). How dual are dual-income couples?: Documenting change from 1970 to 2001. Journal of Marriage and the Family, 68 (1), 11–28.

Raudenbush, S. W. (2001). Comparing personal trajectories and drawing causal inferences from longitudinal data. Annual Review of Psychology, 52(1), 501–525.

Raudenbush, S. W. (2005). How do we study "what happens next"? Annals of the American Academy of Political and Social Science, 602(1), 131–144.

Reichart, E., Chesley, N., & Moen, P. (2007). Beyond the career mystique?: Policies structuring gendered paths in the United States and Germany. Journal of Family Research, 3, 336–369.

Reiss, A. J., Jr. (1989). Ending criminal careers. Washington, DC : MacArthur Foundation and National Institute of Justice.

Reiss, A. J., Jr., & Rhodes, A. L. (1961). The distribution of juvenile delinquency in the social class structure. American Sociological Review, 26(5), 720–732.

Reiss, A. J., Jr., & Roth, J. A. E. (1994). Consequences and control (Vol. 4). Washington, DC : National Academies Press.

Reither, E. N., Hauser, R. M., & Swallen, K. E. (2009). Predicting adult health and mortality from adolescent facial characteristics in yearbook photographs. Demography, 46(1), 27–41.

Rhodes, A. L., Reiss, A. J., Jr., & Duncan, O. D. (1965). Occupational segregation in a metropolitan school system. American Journal of Sociology, 70 (6), 682–694.

Riley, M. W. (1973). Aging and cohort succession: Interpretations and misinterpretations. Public Opinion Quarterly, 37(1), 35–49.

Riley, M. W., Johnson, M. E., & Foner, A. (1972). Aging and society: Vol. 3. A sociology of age stratification. New York: Russell Sage Foundation.

Rimer, S. (2008, October 10). Math skills suffer in U.S. study finds. New York Times, pp. 15, 19.

Rindfuss, R. R., Swicegood, C. G., & Rosenfeld, R. A. (1987). Disorder in the life course: How common and does it matter? American Sociological Review, 52, 785–801.

Rodgers, J. L., St. John, C. A., & Coleman, R. (2005). Did fertility go up after the Oklahoma City bombing?: An analysis of births in metropolitan counties in Oklahoma, 1990–1999. Demography, 42 (4), 675–692.

Rodgers, W. L. (1982). Estimable functions of age, period, and cohort effects. American Sociological Review, 47(6), 774–787.

Rossi, A. S., & Rossi, P. H. (1990). Of human bonding: Parent–child relations across the life course. New York: Aldine.

Rowe, D. C., Jacobson, K. C., & Van den Oord, E. J. C. G. (1999). Genetic and environmental influences on vocabulary IQ: Parental education level as moderator. Child Development, 70 (5), 1151–1162.

Rowlison, R. T., & Felner, R. D. (1988). Major life events, hassles, and adaptation in adolescence: Confounding in the conceptualization and measurement of life stress and adjustment revisited. Journal of Personality and Social Psychology, 55(3), 432–444.

Ruggles, S. (2002). Integrated public use microdata series. Retrieved December 2, 2003, from www.ipums.unm.edu.

Ryder, N. B. (1965). The cohort as a concept in the study of social change. American Sociological Review, 30 (6), 843–861.

Rylander-Rudqvist, T., Hakansson, N., Tybring, G., & Wolk, A. (2006). Quality and quantity of saliva DNA obtained from the self-administrated oragene method—a pilot study on the cohort of Swedish men. Cancer Epidemiology Biomarkers and Prevention, 15(9), 1742–1745.

Sampson, R. J., & Laub, J. H. (1993). Crime in the making: Pathways and turning points through life. Cambridge, MA: Harvard University Press.

Sampson, R. J., & Laub, J. H. (1996). Socioeconomic achievement in the life course of disadvantaged men: Military service as a turning point, circa 1940–1965. American Sociological Review, 61(3), 347–367.

Sampson, R. J., & Laub, J. H. (2003). Life-course desisters?: Trajectories of crime among delinquent boys followed to age 70. Criminology, 41(3), 555–592.

Sampson, R. J., & Laub, J. H. (2005a). A life course view of the development of crime. Annals of the American Academy of Political and Social Science, 602(1), 12–45.

Sampson, R. J., & Laub, J. H. (2005b). Seductions of method: Rejoinder to Nagin and Tremblay's "Developmental trajectory groups: Fact or fiction?" Criminology, 43(4), 905–914.

Sampson, R. J., Laub, J. H., & Eggleston, E. P. (2004a). The aftermath of incarceration in the lives of disadvantaged men: A 50-year follow-up study: Final Report prepared for "The 'Mass' Incarceration Working Group." New York: Russell Sage Foundation.

Sampson, R. J., Laub, J. H., & Eggleston, E. P. (2004b). On the robustness and validity of groups. Journal of Quantitative Criminology, 20 (1), 37–42.

Sampson, R. J., Morenoff, J. D., & Earls, F. (1999). Beyond social capital: Spatial dynamics of collective efficacy for children. American Sociological Review, 64(5), 633–660.

Savla, J., Almeida, D. M., Davey, A., & Zarit, S. H. (2008). Routine assistance to parents: Effects on daily mood and other stressors. Journals of Gerontology B: Psychological Sciences and Social Sciences, 63(3), S154–S161.

Schaeffer, C. M., Petras, H., Ialongo, N., Masyn, K. E., Hubbard, S., Poduska, J., et al. (2006). A comparison of girls' and boys' aggressive–disruptive behavior trajectories across elementary school: Prediction to young adult antisocial outcomes. Journal of Consulting and Clinical Psychology, 74(3), 500–510.

Schauben, L. J., & Frazier, P. A. (1995). Vicarious trauma: The effects on female counselors of working with sexual violence survivors. Psychology of Women Quarterly, 19 (1), 49–64.

Schoen, R., Rogers, S. J., & Amato, P. R. (2006). Wives' employment and spouses' marital happiness: Assessing the direction of influence using longitudinal couple data. Journal of Family Issues, 27(4), 506–528.

Schwalbe, M. L. (1987). On practical and discursive self-knowledge. Humanity and Society, 11, 366–384.

Scott, E. K., London, A. S., & Myers, N. A. (2002). Dangerous dependencies: The intersection of welfare reform and domestic violence. Gender and Society, 16(6), 878–897.

Scott, J., & Alwin, D. (1998). Retrospective versus prospective measurement of life histories in longitudinal research. In J. Z. Giele & G. H. Elder, Jr. (Eds.), Methods of life course research: Qualitative and quantitative approaches (pp. 98–127). Thousand Oaks, CA: Sage.

Segal, D. R., & Segal, M. W. (2004). America's military population. Population Bulletin, 59 (4), 3–40.

Sewell, W. H. (1988). The changing institutional structure of sociology and my career. In M. W. Riley (Ed.), Sociological lives (pp. 119–143). Newbury Park, CA: Sage.

Sewell, W. H., & Armer, J. M. (1966a). Neighborhood context and college plans. American Sociological Review, 31(2), 159–168.

Sewell, W. H., & Armer, J. M. (1966b). Reply to Turner, Michael, and Boyle (On neighborhood context and college plans [I], [II], [III]). American Sociological Review, 31(5), 698–712.

Sewell, W. H., & Armer, J. M. (1972). High school context and college plans: A comment. American Sociological Review, 37(5), 637–639.

Sewell, W. H., Haller, A. O., & Ohlendorf, G. W. (1970). The educational and early occupational status attainment process: Replication and revision. American Sociological Review, 35(6), 1014–1027.

Sewell, W. H., Haller, A. O., & Portes, A. (1969). The educational and early occupational attainment process. American Sociological Review, 34(1), 82–92.

Sewell, W. H., & Hauser, R. M. (1972). Causes and consequences of higher education: Models of the status attainment process. American Journal of Agricultural Economics, 54(6), 851–861.

Sewell, W. H., & Hauser, R. M. (1975). Education, occupation, and earnings: Achievement in the early career. New York: Academic Press.

Sewell, W. H., & Hauser, R. M. (1992). The influence of the American occupational structure on the Wisconsin Model. Contemporary Sociology, 21(5), 598–603.

Sewell, W. H., Hauser, R. M., Springer, K. W., & Hauser, T. S. (2004). As we age: The Wisconsin Longitudinal Study, 1957–2001. In K. Leicht (Ed.), Research in social stratification and mobility (Vol. 20, pp. 3–111). London: Elsevier.

Sewell, W. H., Hauser, R. M., & Wolf, W. C. (1980). Sex, schooling and occupational status. American Journal of Sociology, 86(3), 551–583.

Shanahan, M. J., & Elder, G. H., Jr. (2002). History, agency, and the life course. In L. J. Crockett (Ed.), Agency, motivation, and the life course (pp. 145–185). Lincoln, NE: University of Nebraska Press.

Shanahan, M. J., Erickson, L. D., Vaisey, S., & Smolen, A. (2007). Helping relationships and genetic propensities: A combinatoric study of DRD2, mentoring, and educational continuation. Twin Research and Human Genetics, 10 (2), 285–298.

Shanahan, M. J., & Hofer, S. M. (2005). Social context in gene–environment interactions: Retrospect and prospect. Journals of Gerontology B: Psychological Sciences and Social Sciences, 60, 65–76.

Shanahan, M. J., Hofer, S. M., & Shanahan, L. (2003). Biological models of behavior and the life course. In J. T. Mortimer & M. J. Shanahan (Eds.), Handbook of the life course (pp. 597–622). New York: K luwer Academic/Plenum Press.

Shanahan, M. J., & Macmillan, R. (2007). Biography and the sociological imagination: Contexts and contingencies. New York: Norton.

Shanahan, M. J., Vaisey, S., Erickson, L. D., & Smolen, A. (2008). Environmental contingencies and genetic propensities: Social capital, educational continuation, and a dopamine receptor polymorphism. American Journal of Sociology, 114(S1), S260–S286.

Shavit, Y., & Blossfeld, H.-P. E. (1993). Persistent inequality: Changing educational attainment in thirteen countries. Boulder, CO: Westview Press.

Shuey, K. M., & Willson, A. E. (2008). Cumulative disadvantage and black/white disparities in life-course heath trajectories. Research on Aging, 60 (2), 169–199.

Silverstein, M., Bengston, V. L., & Lawton, L. (1997). Intergenerational solidarity and the structure of adult child–parent relationships in American families. American Journal of Sociology, 103(2), 429–460.

Silverstein, M., & Long, J. D. (1998). Trajectories of grandparents' perceived solidarity with adult grandchildren: A growth curve analysis over 23 years. Journal of Marriage and the Family, 60 (3), 912–923.

Simmons, R. G., Rosenberg, F., & Rosenberg, M. (1973). Disturbance in the self image of adolescence. American Sociological Review, 38 (4), 553–568.

Singer, B., & Ryff, C. D. (2001). Person-centered methods for understanding aging: The integration of numbers and narratives. In R. H. Binstock & L. K. George (Eds.), Handbook of aging and the social sciences (5th ed., pp. 44–65). San Diego: Academic Press.

Singer, J. A. (2004). Narrative identity and meaning making across the adult lifespan: An introduction. Journal of Personality, 72 (3), 437–460.

Singer, J. D., & Willett, J. B. (2003). Applied longitudinal data analysis: Modeling change and event occurrence. New York: Oxford University Press.

Singer, M., Hertas, E., & Scott, G. (2000). Am I my brother's keeper?: A case study of the responsibilities of research. Human Organization, 59 (4), 389–400.

Singley, S. G., & Hynes, K. (2005). Transitions to parenthood. Gender and Society, 19 (3), 376–397.

Slevin, K. F., & Wingrove, C. R. (1998). From stumbling blocks to stepping stones: The life experiences of fifty professional African American women. New York: New York University Press.

Smith, P. H., Tessaro, I., & Earp, J. A. L. (1995). Women's experiences with battering: A conceptualization from qualitative research. Women's Health Issues, 5(4), 173–182.

Sokoloff, N. J., & Dupont, I. (2005). Domestic violence at the intersections of race, class, and gender: Challenges and contributions to understanding violence against marginalized women in diverse communities. Violence Against Women, 11, 38–64.

Soskice, D. (1991). The institutional infrastructure for international competitiveness: A comparative analysis of the U.K. and Germany. In A. B. Atkinson & R. Brunetta (Eds.), Economics for the New Europe: Proceedings of a conference held by the International Economic Association in Venice, Italy, November, 1990 (pp. 45–66). New York: New York University Press.

Spradley, J. P. (1980). Participant observation. New York: Holt, Rinehart & Winston.

Stebbins, R. A. (1972). The unstructured interview as incipient interpersonal relationship. Sociology and Social Research, 56(2), 164–179.

Stolzenberg, R. M. (2001). It's about time and gender: Spousal employment and health. American Journal of Sociology, 107(1), 61–100.

Stone, P. (2007). Opting out?: Why women really quit careers and head home. Berkeley: University of California Press.

Stouffer, S. A., Lumsdaine, A. A., Lumsdaine, M. H., Williams, R. M., Jr., Smith, M. B., Janis, I. L., et al. (1949). The American soldier: Vol. II. Combat and its aftermath. Princeton, NJ: Princeton University Press.

Stouffer, S. A., Suchman, E. A., DeVinney, L. C., Star, S. A., & Williams, R. M., Jr. (1949). The American soldier: Vol. I. Adjustment during army life. Princeton, NJ: Princeton University Press.

Straits, B. C. (1996). Ego-net diversity: Same and cross-sex coworker ties. Social Networks, 18 (1), 29–45.

Straus, M. A. (1992). Children as witnesses to marital violence: A risk factor of lifelong problems among a nationally representative sample of American men and women. In D. F. Schwartz (Ed.), Children and violence: Report of the 23rd Ross Roundtable on Critical Approaches to Common Pediatric Problems (pp. 98–109). Columbus, OH: Ross Laboratories.

Strauss, A. L., & Corbin, J. (1990). Basics of qualitative research: Grounded theory procedures and techniques. Newbury Park, CA: Sage.

Strober, M. H., & Chan, A. M. K. (1999). The road winds uphill all the way: Gender, work, and family in the United States and Japan. Cambridge, MA: MIT Press.

Strohschein, L. (2005). Parental divorce and child mental health trajectories. Journal of Marriage and the Family, 67(5), 1286–1300.

Sweet, S., & Moen, P. (2007). Integrating educational careers in work and family. Community, Work and Family, 10 (2), 231–250.

Taylor, M. G. (2005). Disaggregating disability trajectories: Exploring differences in the disability experience of older adults in the United States. Unpublished dissertation, Duke University, Durham, NC.

Taylor, M. G. (2008). Timing, accumulation and the black/white disability gap in later life: A test of weathering. Research on Aging, 30 (2), 226–250.

Taylor, M. G., & Lynch, S. M. (2004). Trajectories of impairment, social support, and depressive symptoms in later life. Journals of Gerontology B: Psychological Sciences and Social Sciences, 59 (4), S238–S246.

Terman, L. M. (1925). Mental and physical traits of a thousand gifted children. Stanford, CA: Stanford University Press.

Terman, L. M., & Oden, M. H. (1959a). Genetic studies of genius: Vol. 5. The gifted group at mid-life: Thirty-five years of follow-up of the superior child. Stanford, CA: Stanford University Press.

Terman, L. M., & Oden, M. H. (1959b). Genetic studies of genius: Vol. 4. The gifted child grows up: Twenty-five years' follow-up of a superior group. Stanford, CA: Stanford University Press.

Thernstrom, S. (1964). Poverty and progress: Social mobility in a 19th-century city. Cambridge, MA: Harvard University Press.

Thomas, W. I., & Znaniecki, F. (1918–1920). The Polish peasant in Europe and America: Monograph of an immigrant group (Vol. 1–5). Chicago: University of Chicago Press; Boston: Badger Press.

Thompson, L., & Walker, A. J. (1982). The dyad as the unit of analysis: Conceptual and methodological issues. Journal of Marriage and Family, 44(3), 889–900.

Titma, M., & Tuma, N. B. (Eds.). (1995). Paths of a generation: A comparative longitudinal study of young adults in the former Soviet Union. Stanford, CA: Stanford University Press.

Tremblay, R. E., Japel, C., Perusse, D., Mcduff, P., Boivin, M., Zoccolillo, M., et al. (1999). The search for age of "onset" of physical aggression: Rousseau and Bandura revisited. Criminal Behavior and Mental Health, 9 (1), 8–23.

Turnbull, J. E., George, L. K., Landerman, R., Swartz, M. S., & Blazer, D. G. (1990). Social outcomes related to age of onset among psychiatric disorders. Journal of Consulting and Clinical Psychology, 58 (6), 832–839.

Turner, R. H. (1960). Sponsored and contest mobility and the school system. American Sociological Review, 25(6), 855–867.

Turner, R. H. (1964). The social context of ambition. San Francisco: Chandler.

U.S. Department of Health and Human Services, Centers for Disease Control and Prevention. (1988). National Maternal and Infant Health Survey. Retrieved August 14, 2008, from www.cdc.gov/nchs/about/major/nmihs/abnmihs.htm

U.S. Department of Health and Human Services. (1999). Annual update of the Health and Human Services poverty guidelines. Federal Register, 64, 13428–13430.

U.S. Public Health Service. (1980). International classification of diseases, 9th revision, clinical modification. Washington, DC : Author. van de Rijt, A., & Buskens, V. (2006). Trust in intimate relationships: The increased importance of embeddedness for marriage in the United States. Rationality and Society, 18 (2), 123–156.

Verbrugge, L. M., Gruber-Baldini, A. L., & Fozard, J. L. (1996). Age differences and age changes in activities: Baltimore Longitudinal Study of Aging. Journals of Gerontology B: Psychological Sciences and Social Sciences, 51(1), S30–S41.

Vidich, A. J. (1955). Participant observation and the collection and interpretation of data. American Journal of Sociology, 60 (4), 354–360.

Volkart, E. H. (1951). Social behavior and personality: Contributions of W. I. Thomas to theory and social research. New York: Social Science Research Council.

von Eye, A., & Bogat, G. A. (2006). Person-oriented and variable-oriented research: Concepts, results, and development. Merrill–Palmer Quarterly Journal of Developmental Psychology, 52 (3), 390–420.

Wadsworth, M. E. J. (1991). The imprint of time: Childhood, history, and adult life. Oxford, England: Clarendon Press.

Wagmiller, R. L., Jr., Lennon, M. C., Kuang, L., Alberti, P., & Aber, J. L. (2006). The dynamics of economic disadvantage and children's life chances. American Sociological Review, 71(5), 847–866.

Wang, M. (2007). Profiling retirees in the retirement transition and adjustment process: Examining the longitudinal change patterns of retirees' psychological well-being. Journal of Applied Psychology, 92 (2), 455–474.

Warren, J. R., & Halpern-Manners, A. (2007). Is the glass emptying or filling up?: Reconciling divergent trends in high school completion and droput. Educational Researcher, 36(6), 335–343.

Warren, J. R., Sheridan, J. T., & Hauser, R. M. (2002). Occupational stratification across the life course: Evidence from the Wisconsin Longitudinal Study. American Sociological Review, 67(3, June), 432–455.

Wax, R. (1956). Reciprocity as a field technique. Human Organization, 11(3), 34–41.

Weber, M. (1930). The Protestant ethic and the spirit of capitalism (T. Parsons, Trans.). New York: Scribner.

Weinstein, E. A., & Deutschberger, P. (1963). Some dimensions of altercasting. Sociometry, 26(4), 454–466.

Wellman, B., Wong, R. Y.-L., Tindall, D., & Nazer, N. (1997). A decade of network change: Turnover, persistence and stability in personal communities. Social Networks, 19, 27–50.

Wells, T., Sandefur, G. D., & Hogan, D. P. (2004). What happens after the high school years among young persons with disabilities? Social Forces, 82 (2), 803–832.

West, C., & Zimmerman, D.H. (1987). Doing gender. Gender and Society, 1(2), 125–151.

Weyman, A., Heinz, W.R., & Alheit, P. (1996). Society and biography. Paper presented at the Third International Symposium of the Sonderforschungsbereich 186.

Wheaton, B. (1990). Life transitions, role histories, and mental health. American Sociological Review, 55(2), 209–223.

Wheaton, B. (1999). The nature of stressors. In A.V. Horowitz & T.L. Scheid (Eds.), A handbook for the study of mental health: Social contexts, theories, and systems (pp. 176–197). New York: Cambridge University Press.

Wheaton, B., & Clarke, P. (2003). Space meets time: Integrating temporal and contextual influences on mental health in early adulthood. American Sociological Review, 68, 680–706.

White, R.W. (1966). Lives in progress: A study of the natural growth of personality (2nd ed.). New York: Holt, Rinehart & Winston. (Original work published 1952)

Williams, D.R., Lavizzo-Mourney, R., & Warren, R.C. (1994). The concept of race and health status in America. Public Health Reports, 109 (1), 26–41.

Williams, L.A. (2003). Understanding child abuse and violence against women: A life course perspective. Journal of Interpersonal Violence, 18 (4), 441–451.

Willie, C.V. (1988). Commentary on Sociological Lives. In M.W. Riley (Ed.), Sociological lives (Vol. 2, pp. 163–176). Newbury Park, CA: Sage.

Willson, A.E., Shuey, K.M., & Elder, G.H., Jr. (2007). Cumulative advantage processes as mechanisms of inequality in life course health. American Journal of Sociology, 112(6), 1886–1924.

Winship, C., & Morgan, S.L. (1999). The estimation of causal effects from observational data. Annual Review of Sociology, 25, 659–706.

Winston, P., with Angel, R.J., Burton, L.M., Chase-Lansdale, P.L., Cherlin, A.J., Moffitt, R.A., & Wilson, W.J. (1999). Welfare, children, and families: A three-city study. Overview and design. Available online at web.jhu.edu/threecitystudy/images/overviewanddesign.pdf.

Yates, M.E., Tennstedt, S., & Chang, B.H. (1999). Contributors to and mediators of psychological well-being for informal caregivers. Journals of Gerontology B: Psychological Sciences and Social Sciences, 54(1), P12–P22.

Yorgason, J.B., Almeida, D.M., Neupert, S.D., Spiro, A., III, & Hoffman, L. (2006). A dyadic examination of daily health symptoms and emotional well-being in late-life couples. Family Relations, 55(5), 613–624.

Zarit, S.H., & Eggebeen, D.J. (2002). Parent–child relationships in adulthood and later years. In M.H. Bornstein (Ed.), Handbook of parenting (2nd ed., Vol. 1, pp. 135–161). Mahwah, NJ: Erlbaum.

Zautra, A.J. (2003). Emotions, stress, and health. New York: Oxford University Press.

Zautra, A.J., Finch, J.F., Reich, J.W., & Guarnaccia, C.A. (1991). Predicting the everyday life events of older adults. Journal of Personality, 59 (3), 507–538.

Zimmer, Z., & House, J.S. (2003). Education, income and functional limitation transitions among American adults: Contrasting onset and progression. International Journal of Epidemiology, 32 (6).

4 Gender as the Next Top Model of Global Consumer-Citizenship

Lindsay Palmer

At first she looks like a transient, slouching in an alley. Her hair is disheveled, her face dirty, and her clothing in disarray. But the sudden flashing of a photographer's bulb suggests otherwise. The Manhattan alley in which she poses looks too clean and the people ambling by her look too well dressed. From a hidden corner, a director's voice calls for tears, demanding that this fashion model deliver an emotionally-charged performance of homelessness. Behind her, real transients dressed in haute couture enjoy their quite temporary makeovers. The bulbs flash, the girls pose, and their diverse stories are streamlined into spectacle.

In this photo shoot for the CW Television Network's hit program, 'America's Next Top Model,' panic is the spectacle being captured on film. Yet, this is not the flashy panic of the Hollywood horror picture, or even the private panic of an individual living on the streets. This is instead moral panic, a visceral social reaction to the dissolution of the nation state, fueled by neoliberal politics and exacerbated by a diverse array of television genres. The globalization of these media plays a key role in engendering such moral panic, as stabilized constructs of culture give way to what an open-ended culture of homelessness (Morley, 2000). Morley interweaves the notion of home with the concept of nation, explaining how both have destabilized due to increased physical mobility and the globalization of new communication technologies, "which routinely transgress the symbolic boundaries around both the private household and the nation state" (p. 3).

The home has long operated as a site for identity construction in the US as a zone demarcated by boundaries that designate an inside and an outside and who belongs there. The home has also served as a prime space in which consumption occurs, whether it is the necessary consumption of food or the culturally driven consumption of glistening appliances like the Frigidaire. This home space and its important functions have been assigned a feminine quality both on the smaller level of the suburban house safeguarded by a conscientious wife and mother figure, as well as on the level of national rhetoric, where the home is recast as a feminized nation in need of protection. Because of its originally strict boundaries, the feminized home-space has, throughout US history, been conceptualized as an immobile and stable space. Yet, as Morley (2000) asserts, these boundaries are dissolving, aligning consumption and identity construction with the more fluid demands of globalization.

Programs like 'America's Next Top Model' interrogate the transgression of such boundaries in surprising ways, thematically aligning gender performance with the American concept of home, and celebrating mobility—liberated womanhood—while simultaneously fortifying that womanhood's borders. Such contradictions are far from novel, as Cady (2006) argues. Cady traces this phenomenon back to the medieval era when women were characterized as "supposedly passive, yet potentially powerful" as transgressive entities that "therefore must be carefully monitored and contained" (p. 17). Cady also explains how, in a period when money was viewed with deep suspicion, the writers of the era would conflate portrayals of women with portrayals of money, implying that women served as "items of exchange because of some aspect of their nature," which was considered just as capricious as the nature of money itself (p. 27). In other words, the medieval era saw its own moral panic over the purportedly dual nature of women as well as over the new currency that was thought to be capable of transgressing the boundaries of the old land-based systems even as it was also viewed as impotent in the face of powerful masculinist and classist traditions.

Current US television programs continue to conceptually conflate women with money, positing them as powerful yet dangerous subjects who must also learn to become commodities for exchange in an era where commodities themselves transgress national boundaries and reorganize cultural communities. Through the technology of the makeover contest, *America's Next Top Model* posits the space inside the borders that demarcate femininity—even the "liberated" femininity of the postfeminist age—as a destination to which all women must attempt to arrive. 'America's Next Top Model' is both a contest program and a traditional makeover program; its characters undergo physical and psychological refashioning, covertly encouraging the same transformation in the program's viewers, who also encounter this phenomenon in news programs as well as soap operas, sitcoms, and game shows (Heller, 2006). Heller (2006) attributes the increasing popularity of the makeover to the twenty-first century political climate, drawing on Gates's assertion that "the traditional importance of home, the post-September 11th hunger for security, and a growing middle class sense of entitlement" all combine to create a huge potential audience of diverse individuals eager to write new personal narratives that guarantee them a stable home within an increasingly borderless society (p. 2).

Despite its supposed interest in individualization, 'America's Next Top Model' has a specific agenda for each contestant, and arguably each viewer's newly fashioned narrative. From the Bronx native undergoing therapy for anger management to the Somalian immigrant overcoming the trauma of female circumcision, the women of 'America's Next Top Model' are encouraged to enhance their differences, with the result that they take better photographs and glamorize the television program with their inevitable conflicts. In this sense, 'America's Next Top Model' centers personal narrative on the notion of consumption, giving the illusion of individualization while simultaneously streamlining difference into a coherent model narrative. This model not only teaches Americans how to be good global consumers, but it also tells a story of global citizenship that cultural theorists have explored at length, with varying results. I will delineate the quite different arguments of Seyla Benhabib (2002), Néstor García Canclini (2001), and Toby Miller (2007), in hopes of underscoring the ways in which the interactions between cultures reinforce the erasure of 'culture' and 'citizenship' as stabilized concepts that link notions of belonging with notions of home. I will then complicate these theorists' frameworks, showing how gender's connection with the concept of home informs the reconceptualization of belonging in a globalized era. 'America's Next Top Model' will serve as my example of this reconceptualization, propagating narratives of empowering female mobility while still policing the boundaries of gender in a way that posits femininity as the universal home to which all modern women belong.

MODEL NARRATIVES

In her book *The Claims of Culture*, Benhabib (2002) compellingly refutes the idea of culture as a coherent home, yet she fails to grasp the universalizing implications of her own argument, positing a purportedly impartial and democratic public sphere as a space in which women from all cultural origins can write and rewrite their personal narratives at will. Benhabib defines cultures as "complex human practices of signification and representation . . . which are internally riven by conflicting narratives" (p. ix). In other words, Benhabib argues that rather than existing as discrete entities with original starting-points, cultures are formed through complex dialogue with other cultures. This dialogue depends on the notion of narrative. Benhabib (2002) explains that cultures present themselves through narrative because human actions and relations are, as a rule, formed through a "double hermeneutic: we identify *what* we do through an *account* of what we do" (p. 6). These complex cultural narratives are always in flux as a result of interaction with conflicting narratives. Because of this, Benhabib calls for an impartial public space where cultures can struggle for recognition and even rewrite themselves without danger of domination.

At the heart of this notion is Benhabib's (2002) "norm of universal respect," which stipulates that every speaking, rational creature has equal right to participate in the conversation (p. 14). Benhabib asserts that maintaining the impartiality of this sphere, as well as the norm of universal respect on which discourse depends is the task of democracy. Thus, Benhabib separates the notion of the individual from the notion of culture. With these rights understood, Benhabib (2002) claims that a democratic model would generate a safe and productive space where complex cultures could write and rewrite their defining narratives and where individuals could break with these narratives in order to write narratives of their own.

Benhabib (2002) derives her notion of the impartial public sphere from the work of Jürgen Habermas, who, like Benhabib, emphasizes rationality and universalism. Yet, it is this tendency toward universalism that masks the inequalities which have always existed in the formation of the public sphere, which in the 18th century excluded women as well as anyone who was not white or of the bourgeois class. Sakai (1997) explains that Habermas attributes this purportedly impartial space to the "rational" and modern west, which he posits as a concrete and even ubiquitous entity (p. 155). While Habermas decisively asserts his epistemological arguments with an outcome being reinvigorated trust in universalism, Sakai (1997) on the other hand, argues that proponents of universalism often use its rhetoric to rationalize and influence social institutions, while simultaneously veiling the fact that universalism serves as a "strategy of dominance by the most advanced particularity" (pp. 157–158).

This reading of Habermas complicates Benhabib's (2002) optimistic delineation of the new ways in which cultures can write and rewrite themselves in a world where old notions of belonging are dissolving. Benhabib's tendency to mimic Habermas's universalizing rhetoric covers over the inequalities embedded in that rhetoric, even as she claims to conceptualize a space in which women of all nations can write their own stories. In other words, Benhabib puts too much faith in the universal power of narrative, as Kompridis (2006) affirms. In other words, Benhabib puts too much faith in the universal power of narrative, attributing to it culture, subjective formation, and institutionally inscribed social codes of behavior (Kompridis, 2006). If we looked at narrative from this angle, we would encounter "not a quasi-transcendental account of normative legitimacy, but a historical narrative of legitimation" (Kompridis, 2006, p. 392). This legitimation always serves the most advanced particularity, rather than successfully serving the "humankind" that proves to be far too multifarious for one such term to properly represent. Such an observation points to the manipulative power of narrative to override other narratives; it also points to Benhabib's failure to adequately account for one example of this manipulation, which is the narrative of globalization as modernizing social structure rather than economic strategy. While Benhabib (2002) does speak of the "global interdependence" of meaning and interpretation in the face of globalization, she does not discuss the ways in which consumption drives this interdependence, but rather focuses only on the narratives, citing the opinion that "our agency consists in our capacity to weave out of those narratives our individual life stories" (p. 15).

US reality programs like 'America's Next Top Model' also put too much faith in the universal power of the life story, mirroring Benhabib's (2002) claim for narrative agency, and promoting the notion that the conflict between already existing individualities and their milieu ultimately leads to healthier subjectivities. The contradictions between such universalism and the personal narratives that universalism purportedly protects surface in the program's tendency to refer to its contestants on a first-name basis, manufacturing the personalized intimacy between cast members and viewers that Leppert and Wilson (2008) trace in other reality TV programs, while simultaneously reducing each woman to one name, flashing at the bottom of the screen. The opening to the program also functions this way, demanding: "What is beauty to you?" and setting the tone for the contestants to draw on past and present experiences in order to make themselves universally beautiful. For example, the contestant named Fatima cites her experience with female circumcision, explaining that she wants to be a spokesperson for other women who have suffered the same assault on their bodies. She also employs her knowledge of homelessness during the Manhattan photo-shoot, reminiscing on how the children she once knew in Somalia made fun of her for living in a shelter. Following Tyra Banks' instruction to "study yourself and find what is strong and different and interesting," Fatima employs her personal narrative to fashion herself into the aesthetic ideal touted by the most advanced particularity safeguarding the purportedly impartial space of the American public sphere.

Just as Benhabib (2002) claims that democracy safeguards this public sphere, so 'America's Next Top Model' claims to safeguard it, even when one such life story clashes with another. For example, Fatima's process of self-realization collides with that of Marvita, an African-American woman from the Bronx. She, like Fatima, has experienced homelessness, yet this and African ancestry is really all that she and Fatima have in common. "I've never met a mean African," she tells Fatima in one of their many arguments on the program. The two contestants fight about each other's diction, about each other's tone of voice, and about each other's way of handling personal trauma. After arguing heatedly for a few episodes, they reach an understanding that results in the revision of their earlier thoughts on each other. Fatima comes to understand that Marvita's brusqueness is due to her growing up in the Bronx, warding off lascivious relatives as well as violent peers. In turn, Marvita accepts (despite her inability to fully understand) Fatima's circumcision, as well as her particular experience with homelessness. In this sense, 'America's Next Top Model' seems to encourage the sort of contestation and even confrontation that Benhabib (2002) says occurs because of cultural interdependence in a globalized world. Both Fatima and Marvita are encouraged to embrace and revise their unique narratives, yet to respect each other's differences as being equally valid.

Yet, these narratives are highly mediated by the most advanced particularity that wields power over what is finally revealed as a mere simulation of an already flawed public sphere. Indeed, the program's producers and the fashion industry gurus who influence them take a special interest in narratives centered on race, encouraging the contestants to embrace and yet transform the racial origin with which they feel most inclined to identify. For example, Brittany of cycle eleven identifies herself as being half African-American and half American Indian. "My ethnicity and my racial background, it is special to me. But I'm a diverse person. I want to appeal to everybody," she says. Similarly, contestant Sheena announces that she is half Japanese and half Korean, but that she likes "all colors and all flavors." While the judges routinely celebrate the interaction of differing racial narratives, they especially approve of contestants who stand ready to forget those narratives, at least for one photo shoot. This ability to embody rather than simply appreciate diversity not only proves crucial to remaining in the competition, it also reveals the ways in which Sakai's notion of the most advanced particularity comes into play, influencing what masquerades as an impartial space for discourse. The program producers and the fashion industry serve as this advanced particularity, always getting the final say in which types of racial narratives are most easily marketed. Ultimately, Banks teaches the women how to impersonate any conceivable aspect of femininity, engendering images that cut across racially oriented lines.

If the contestants cannot achieve this—if they stick out, in other words, in ways that Banks fears will not sell the clothing—they are eliminated. "I don't want another bitchy black girl on this show," Banks tells one contestant, simultaneously stereotyping her and paradoxically demanding that she step outside of stereotype and into a universalized notion of femininity. Later, Banks approvingly tells a white contestant that her new makeover causes her to appear 'racially ambiguous,' enabling little girls from all ethnic backgrounds to see themselves in this contestant. In turn, these little girls are expected to buy the clothing displayed on the model with whom they purportedly relate, actualizing their own burgeoning sense of self through consumption. In this sense, the program producers propagate the show's acceptance of diversity, even as they demand that such diversity be streamlined into universally marketable expressions of personal narrative.

The one narrative that 'America's Next Top Model' contestants are not expected to revise, however, is the narrative that constructs and employs gender to define and even safeguard the sphere in which the contestants operate. While the program is produced and the contest judged by straight and queer-identified men and women of varying ethnicities, the contestants must all be read as female, whatever their racial identity or sexual orientation. In this sense, the subjectivities they fashion and re-fashion for themselves must maintain one crucial facet: They are 'women,' teaching other women how to clothe their bodies and, thus, fuel the fashion industry. Such womanhood is constantly implied, from the show's opening question, "What is beauty to you?" to Banks' tireless demand for the women to "fiercely" embrace their femininity. While Banks encourages girls like Fatima to overcome long histories of gender-based abuse, she ultimately expects that Fatima create a new femininity that will in turn set a standard for potential female consumers. Banks expects the same of Marvita, who must overcome her inability to be close to others in order to take believable pictures. Since Marvita's unemotional exterior is a direct result of her sexual abuse, Banks encourages Marvita to face this past and overcome it, restoring a sense of sentimentality that will show on film. At the very least, Banks demands the appearance of feminine conventionality from her contestants.

In this sense, the sphere of contestation simulated by this program actually serves as what Berlant (2002) calls an 'intimate public,' rather than a counter-public or all-inclusive primary public sphere. Such publics "fuse feminine rage and feminist rage . . . hailing the wounded to testify, to judge, to yearn, and to think beyond the norms of sexual difference, a little" (Berlant, 2002, p. 1). The contestants on 'America's Next Top Model' are not always angels in the reality show house, they are not all white or middle class, and they do not always sexually desire men. Yet, they do all "love the conventionality" of their gender, and as Berlant (2002) puts it, they see such conventionality as a way of negotiating belonging, rather than as a constraint (p. 3). They see such conventionality as a shared home. Such a portrayal of womanhood in turn implies a similar sense of belonging for the female viewers rooting for Marvita and Fatima, who internalize the rhetoric of transformation. The very notion of transformation, of transforming yet still embodying femininity, suggests the pleasure of such belonging while paradoxically suggesting the freedom to operate outside the boundaries of the outdated and constrictive norms of femininity—'a little.'

The inherent 'littleness' of this margin of freedom becomes evident in cycle eleven, when a new contestant reveals to the other women that she is, in fact, a pre-op transgender. "Personally, I prefer 'born in the wrong body,'" Isis explains to the camera and her implied viewers, "meaning I was born physically male . . . but everything else about me was female." Isis also finds herself explaining her situation to the judges, as well as the other contestants. Almost every time the camera is pointed her way, in fact, Isis must rearticulate her story, the familiar "born in the wrong body" narrative, as if in awareness of the slipperiness of the narratives that both free her and constrain her. "It's not something I chose," Isis says. "It's just who I always been [sic]." Such an assertion appeases the curiosity of some of the contestants and thrills Banks, who asserts that she first noticed Isis posing in the background of the transient-themed photo shoots of cycle ten. "This girl [was] absolutely amazing," Banks says, pointing to an emotionally-charged photo of Isis hovering behind the cycle ten contestant. Because of this photo, Banks explains that she called Isis to audition for cycle eleven, fully accepting Isis' drive to belong, not only to the fashion industry, but to 'women's culture' in general.

Isis's desire to belong, to find a home in the conventionality of the term 'woman,' haunts this season as her image haunts the contestants' image in the photo from cycle ten. Yet, not everyone accepts her. One contestant named Kacey asks Isis, "Ain't this supposed to be a girl competition? How did you get through the door?" Another contestant tells the camera: "If I have to get along with Isis I will, but then again, if it comes between me and my goal. . . I'll stomp that man right outta' the competition." This same contestant, incidentally sporting the name of Clark, confides in contestant Hannah that she is afraid of getting into the swimming pool with Isis. She justifies her view by claiming that she is not close-minded—she is simply traditional. "You walk around like that in a small town, you'll get shot," Clark says, criminalizing Isis's perceived homelessness, her inability to conform fully to the conventionality of gender. The problem Clark seems to have with Isis is that her transgression is more than a 'little' one. Clark grins at her own boyish name and easily kisses another girl in the hot tub, playing into the program's theme of liberated and transformed femininity. Yet, she cannot allow someone whose body does not reflect her own to have a home in the intimate public she shares with others who identify with the term 'woman.' Since Isis does not start out a 'woman,' in the view of many of the contestants, since she must transform her body as well as her subjectivity, she is not finally resignifying femininity, but is instead masquerading as female.

Despite the contestants' suspicions, the 'America's Next Top Model' judges assert that a model has to be "many different things to many people," implying that a model must become a master-storyteller, able to obscure any perceived origin in order to embody an image that will then provide the viewer with a large selection of consumerist options from which to choose. This assertion echoes Haug's (1986) theory of the aesthetic innovation which regenerates demand, convincing the consumer that the newest commodity is the most essential (pp. 43–44). In this sense, the judges search for contestants who can successfully change their own image into the 'newest thing,' aligning that image with the clothing that will then entice the consumer. As Redden (2007) explains, this drive for reality television contestants to fashion and refashion themselves is consistent with contemporary social theory in which emphasis is on hyper-individualism. Redden (2007) traces the theory that 'being right' no longer equates with following custom, but rather with choosing the 'right' commodities from a wide selection (p. 157). According to Redden (2007), reality TV cast members draw on different readings of uniqueness in order to serve as "typifications of individuality" not necessarily dependent upon stabilized notions of culture (p. 156). In makeover television, all participants are ultimately propelled from their unique origins toward moral consumerism, where the morality relies on the individual's ability to make good consumerist choices based on a plethora of options. 'America's Next Top Model' propels its contestants in the same way, first demanding that the contestants become good consumer-citizens and then expecting them to properly model such consumerism in order to encourage it in the program's viewers. By exploring this aspect of the program, I will reveal the ways in which the empowering narratives of female mobility align with the perceived mobility of currency itself, positioning these contestants and the female viewers who internalize their messages as consumers and commodities paradoxically connected to both the western concept of home and the Western fear of homelessness.

AESTHETIC INNOVATION AND REFASHIONING THE SELF

The title of this program, 'America's Next Top Model,' points to its consumerist focus even without the assistance of the blatant product placement designed to look like 'gifts' that the contestants must then properly enjoy. In cycle ten, for instance, the contestants hear a knock on the door of their loft and run into the foyer to find an array of high-end handbags and Apple Bottom jeans. Some of the contestants immediately begin to change into their new clothes. Others conspicuously carry their handbags everywhere they travel for the rest of the season. However, some of the contestants fail to make use of these gifts as well as the fashion advice they receive while on the show. When Kim, of cycle ten, approaches the judges' panel wearing a headband with a large ribbon, the judges laugh and poke fun at her. They then demand that she take the headband off. "Ooooh girl, this outfit," Tyra clucks disapprovingly. The mild disapproval of the judges and the other contestants turns into scorn, though, when Kim announces that she is no longer interested in modeling such expensive clothing, as she personally finds it ridiculous to pay $2000 for a single outfit. "Kim wants to model because it's pretty and blah-blah-blah," derides Fatima. "Maybe this is not the right place for her." Since she fails to align her individuality with the principles of proper consumption, Kim quickly leaves the program.

Isis also experiences this crash course in proper consumerism. When she approaches the judges' panel in poorly-matched clothing, her hair in disarray, the judges tell her she looks 'common.' They then inform Isis that when she faces them at panel each week, she must look like a model, yet what Banks and the other judges imply in this scene is that Isis must look like a female model. Her hair must appear soft and controlled, and her clothing must accentuate her figure, enabling her to serve as the object of the desiring male gaze, as well as the studious female gaze. No mention is made of Isis's biological structure at this panel session; instead, she is fully accepted as someone who has eschewed her perceived origin and who is now writing a new story that must align with the model narrative propagated by this television program. In this sense, Isis's personal narrative engenders the model narrative that anyone and everyone can write his or her own story with a little help from certain clothing lines.

From this angle, then, 'America's Next Top Model' seems to mirror Canclini's (2001) global "model of society in which many state functions have disappeared or been assumed by private corporations, and in which social participation is organized through consumption rather than through the exercise of citizenship" (p. 5). Unlike Benhabib (2002), Canclini explores the interaction between consumption and citizenship rather than simply exploring the global interdependence of cultures in the face of global change. He states that now citizenship is based on "the private consumption of commodities and media offerings rather than abstract rules of democracy" (Canclini, 2001, p. 5). Viewing consumption through this lens, Canclini cites the disappearance of stable concepts like "culture" and "nation," arguing that we instead inhabit an era of fragmentation and hybridity, where identity groups are formed according to codes other than those of ethnic or cultural origin. Now those codes serve as "mobile pacts for the interpretation of commodities and messages," enabling the formation of international communities founded on patterns of consumption (Canclini, 2001, pp. 43–44).

The contestants of 'America's Next Top Model' at first seem to represent just this sort of 'international' community, founded on the shared consumption of haute couture (or strategic knockoffs) as well as on the shared consumption of female empowerment slogans such as 'Dare to be fierce,' and 'What is beauty to you?' Gender plays a crucial role in the formation of such communities, especially when the commodities in question contribute to the construction of a purportedly "international" version of femininity. In order for this community to truly seem international, the producers of this American program employ racial narrative even as the English language and the white standard of 'racial ambiguity' underscores this community's notion of womanhood. Meanwhile, 'America's Next Top Mode' has engendered several counterparts in varying countries, some of which fuse the 'fierce' femininity and the 'racial ambiguity' of the American program with televisual techniques more specific to each particular region in which this programming appears. For example, the opening of 'China's Next Top Model, Brazil's Next Top Model,' and 'Russia's Next Top Model' (also referred to as 'You are a Supermodel') all feature the same aggressive music with sexualized shots of each contestant gazing fiercely into the camera, propagating the western fashion industry's version of femininity as the globally accepted version, from Shanghai to Moscow.

While 'America's Next Top Model' certainly illuminates the ways in which cultural identity is now often founded on consumption rather than on the concept of nation, this program reduces culture to the mise-en-scène which Canclini (2001) attempts to dismantle, transforming what he views as a montage of multiple viewpoints into a coherent whole that serves a distinct purpose. In this sense, US television programming is certainly not contributing to the new perspective that Canclini propagates despite the fact that it is overflowing national boundaries and influencing other programming traditions, even as European and Latin American entertainment television overflows US boundaries and sometimes influences the content and style of programs at 'home.' Thus, the consumption-driven fluidity of which Canclini speaks does not necessarily lead to the fragmentation of universalized narratives, but instead may only lead to reductive revisions of these narratives that are employed by the most advanced particularity existing within various cultural groups. In other words, US television takes culture and pieces what Canclini (2001) terms the "effervescent montage of discontinuous images" (p. 84), into a quite continuous image, a recognizable home.

'America's Next Top Model' at first seems to create this image of home through its rather nationalist tendency to flood each episode with establishing shots of the US city in which the contest is taking place. In cycle ten, the contestants live in Manhattan, and each week their dramatic conflicts occur only after an establishing shot of Manhattan flashes onto the screen. These shots show a financial Manhattan: Times Square, Rockefeller Plaza, and the Empire State Building, reinforcing one distinct map of New York, the "all-American" map of a booming business center integral to the progress of the global north. The model narrative of individualization in this program, then, is interwoven with a limiting visual rhetoric, suggesting the important influence of the global north and its corporations on this notion of consumer-citizenship. Connell (2007) asserts that social theory "sees and speaks" from the global north, employing globalization to "name-the-world-as-a-whole" as its object of knowledge (p. 368). This tendency likely stems from the same impulse that prompts 'America's Next Top Model' producers to similarly objectify this world-as-a-whole as the proverbial home that belongs to everyone and to which everyone belongs in the moment of no longer belonging. Thus, what Morley (2000) describes as our seemingly disconnected culture from a fixed home becomes a rhetorical tool, veiling its own use of the same monolithic logic that underpins the notion of belonging, the notion of domesticity, and the notion of proper consumption that occurs within that space.

This 'culture of homelessness' is reflected alongside monolithic notions of home in cycle ten of 'America's Next Top Model,' when the contestants pose as homeless people on the streets of Manhattan. Within the space of a North American metropolis, the contestants enact the moment of belonging through no longer belonging; they pose as people with no stabilized identity. Yet, they are all recognizably female, posing on a freshly constructed set rather than in an alley and mimicking a photo of Tyra Banks dressed as a transient, holding a sign that reads: 'Will pose for change.' This image again invokes the dangerous fluidity of the feminine and the financial while simultaneously attempting to contain that fluidity by assigning it a specific narrative within the simulated space for discourse that appears on the television screen; the money itself remains hidden, the alley remains suspiciously clean, and the contestants themselves are carefully contained within the space of the photographic and televisual frames. As Morley (2000) suggests, the notion of cleanliness often coincides with notions of secured boundaries or national homogeneity. This process operates at the familial and societal level, implying that "the family may of course be mobile as it moves through this threatening, external world, but its boundaries must remain secure" (Morley, 2000, p. 141).

   While the notion of gender, like the notion of culture and nationhood, is represented in this program as an entity in flux, the word 'woman' still remains intact. The contestants and the members of the consumption-based community this program creates are expected to hold to the notion of womanhood in order to remain part of this community. Thus, while the word 'woman shifts and morphs and appears to cross boundaries to defy notions of home, it actually serves as a home on the move in the same way that a 'nation' without geographic borders may continue to police its philosophical and political borders, even as it travels throughout and attempts to infiltrate the world. In this sense, gender and nation work together to dictate the structures of Canclini's (2001) international communities, generating consumer-citizens who pursue their own fashioning and their new sense of belonging in true neoliberal spirit. It is this neoliberal agenda that Miller (2007) argues contributes to the real fashioning of citizens, as a reaction to what he calls the "crisis of belonging" that occurs due to the disintegration of nations and cultures in the face of globalization (p. 1). Through Miller's lens, I will explain how neoliberalism constructs notions of home around an 'inside/outside' binary. I will then show that, especially through the technology of television, neoliberalism solidifies this same inside/outside binary in relation to gender as it simultaneously facilitates the mobilization of gender as commodity.

INSIDE AND OUTSIDE

While the rhetoric of homelessness permeates the globalized world, real homelessness or "not-belonging," often results in legal action against the material bodies that represent this problem (Morley, 2000, p. 26). Since citizenship has traditionally relied not solely on the notion of rootedness, but also on the notion of property ownership, the transients who cannot even give a mailing address to prospective employers are constantly relocated and, thus, made invisible. In the same way, those identities not traditionally thought to belong in certain nations experience a similar, though rhetorical relocation. The 'crisis of belonging' is realigned alongside the problematic discourse of multiculturalism or a self-contradictory model of individualization on a reality television show. This underscores Garland's (2008) assertion that the Western media tend to reduce the mobilizing effects of moral panic. In other words, while some moral panics can cause "the deviance in question" to be "amplified or altogether transformed," the inner workings of the media that exacerbate such panics tend to inhibit positive transformation (Garland, 2008, pp. 7, 10). Thus, even as programs like 'America's Next Top Model' propagate narratives of increased mobility, they actually decrease the mobility of the truly transformative discourses that moral panic could productively produce, obscuring the reality of difference behind a universalizing rhetoric of collectively 'not-belonging' that still implies the importance of belonging to a particular identity group.

This contradiction is not unique to reality television, but also appears in the U.S. news media's commentary on the 'crisis of belonging.' Miller's (2007) work explores the ways in which this crisis "is both registered and held in check in US news programming" (p. 1). Echoing the news media's famous mantra, Miller claims that the crisis of belonging is a crisis of 'who, what, when, and where,' and he cites the drive to belong, as well as the sense of not belonging, as a product of the appropriation of culture by a neoliberal project that eclipses the power of the traditional 'American' state. Like Canclini (2001), Miller (2007) situates the formation of identity around consumption, arguing that "with consumers targeted by a culture-driven economy, their identities come to be points of sociopolitical and commercial organization" (p. 9). In other words, the notions that have always been closely connected with the concept of universalized identity origin, or 'home'—access to food and protection from 'outsiders'—all become commodities manipulated by the mass media, pointing again to the ways in which the concept of home generates a site for identity construction and the consumption so important to that construction.

Miller (2007) first delineates the ways in which television manipulates notions of 'inside' and 'outside,' 'secure,' and 'endangered' in the US. He outlines how, during and directly after the September 11th attacks on the World Trade Center, the US news media "set a premium on the lives of Manhattan residents," indicating their "inside" status while simultaneously labeling certain groups both within and outside the US as terrorists (Miller, 2007, p. 107). He recounts how journalists during this time were instructed to be "patriots first, and journalists second," revealing another important trait of belonging: loyalty to the community to which one belongs (Miller, 2007, pp. 99, 107). Morley (2000) states that in order to possess a home— "the natural place of shelter where we can lock the doors against misfortune and unwanted outsiders"—one must often adhere to a rigid set of requirements decided upon by all who occupy the home space (p. 18). In the case of September 11th, journalists not only adhered; they helped create the requirements. Morley explains how US and European broadcasting has always created a national sense of unity by bringing events from which many viewers would be excluded into their homes and thus giving them the illusion of inclusion. During and directly after September 11th, this occurred in the negative sense, bringing carefully chosen images of infiltration into American homes. These images were coupled with patriotic symbols, such as flags and soldiers, contributing to an oppressive culture of national group-think Berlant (2008). In this sense, journalists tried to create a homogenous notion of home that necessarily posited certain types of difference as dangerous. This sense of danger led to the intentional transgression of regional and legal boundaries by US authorities, hence the attacks on Afghanistan and Iraq and the imprisonments in Guantánamo Bay (Miller, 2007).

While journalism works with precision to create these notions of inside and outside, entertainment television constructs its own "inside/outside" binaries in just as insidious a fashion. Ouellette (2009) posits this as an issue of governmentality, tracing James Hay's argument that television facilitates the internalization of self-governance since the neoliberal agenda depends on government deregulation in order to transgress national boundaries and institute current corporate practices; incidentally, neoliberal rhetoric also seeks to avoid government involvement in the life of the individual who must make herself over into the ideal consumer-citizen. Ouellette adds that a long tradition of feminist discourse locates this self-governance in the make-over tradition so ubiquitous to western reality television programming.

I would like to conceptualize how, through the technology of the make-over, US entertainment television connects such governance with the inside/outside binary, positioning the 'inside' status as a destination to which all women must dutifully attempt to arrive, even as that 'inside' status over-flows national boundaries and materializes at multiple sites. 'America's Next Top Model' particularly points to the ways in which such refashioning is structured around complex notions of inside and outside that are explic-itly tied to gender. Isis serves as both outsider and insider in the same epi-sode, depending on which cast member is speaking at the time. Both Banks's approval of Isis and the contestants' disapproval work in the same way. Isis's constantly shifting status helps solidify the category, the stable home that each contestant finds in gender. In this sense, Isis recognizes herself as outsider, trying to get inside and achieving this journey inside through a suc-cessful embodiment of the mobile image of femininity.

The proper maintenance of this image of femininity depends on another trait coiled within the concept of home: access to food. Miller (2007) explains how food is the basis of the earliest class systems, symbolizing consumption and signifying one's particular caliber of home within the national home. The US interest in food has led to what Miller (2007) calls "Food TV . . . a key site of risk and moral panic, a space that forms and maintains citizens" (p. 121). This formation of citizenship manifests itself in "mobilized rhetoric of neoliberal self-governance," which blames obe-sity on poor consumer choices rather than on poor food regulation (Miller, 2007, p. 122). On 'America's Next Top Model,' proper consumption of food products leads to proper formation of woman as commodity. Because of this, the show's judges and contestants often address each other's eating habits. In cycle four, for instance, the judges constantly attack the contestant Keenyah for her purported weight gain. Accordingly, the cameras follow the woman around the contestants' apartment, capturing close-ups of every-thing she eats, yet cycles nine and ten each champion their token 'plus-sized model,' asserting the beauty of womanly curves, and carefully capturing those same close-up shots of potato pancakes and peanut butter bars. When one of the plus-sized models begins to lose weight, she is eliminated from the contest as abruptly as the standard model that the judges chastise for gaining weight. In both instances, the contestants are punished for failing to serve as a model of proper self-governance. Through this visual rhetoric, woman is again invoked as the powerful, yet capricious entity, a commodity for exchange that is expected to know and enhance her own commodity value.

This phenomenon serves as a prime example of Miller's (2007) assertion that subjectivities are manipulated and identities produced through the neoliberal project that utilizes moral panic and the identity crises informing such panic in order to achieve its goal. 'America's Next Top Model' draws on the rhetoric of self-governance in a way that at first seems to suggest autonomy in the fashioning of personal narrative. Yet, at the end of every episode, this autonomy is replaced with explicit instructions for self-transformation, courtesy of Tyra Banks and her lackeys. While the instructions differ from contestant to contestant, implying the 'plethora of options' which Redden (2007) attributes to globalization, the contestants are still expected to make the correct choices in order to achieve the sanctioned sort of success, predicated on their adherence to gender rules. The women are expected to find and employ "consumer options that satisfy and personalize differentiated notions of value" (Redden, 2007, p. 151). However, they are also expected to make the choices that will transform them into role-models for the millions of female viewers eyeing both the bodies and the clothing from the home-space of their sofas. Camouflaged as entertainment, 'America's Next Top Model' employs the theme of homelessness to read the mobility that defies social constructs like 'nation' and 'culture,' while simultaneously masking the immobility of gender. Gender, in all its shifting shapes, paradoxically becomes a site for belonging and no-longer-belonging, an articulation of homelessness, and the last home standing.

REFERENCES

Benhabib, S. (2002). *The claims of culture: Equality and diversity in the global l era*. Princeton, NJ: Princeton UP.

Berlant, L. (2008). *The female complaint: The unfinished business of sentimentality in American culture*. Durham, NC: Duke UP.

Cady, D. (2006). The gender of money. *Genders, 44*. Retrieved from http://www.genders.org/g44/g44_cady.html

Canclini, N. G. (2001). *Consumers and citizens*. Minneapolis: UM Press.

Connell, R. (2007). The Northern theory of globalization. *Sociological Theory, (25)*4, 368–385. Retrieved from http://googlescholar.com.

CW Television Network. (2006-present). *America's next top model*. UPN.

Garland, D. (2008). On the concept of moral panic. *Crime, media, and culture, (4)*1, 9–30. Retrieved from http://sagepub.com.

Haug, W. (1986). *Critique of commodity aesthetics: Appearance, sexuality, and advertising in capitalist society*. Cambridge: Polity.

Heller, D. (Ed.). (2007). *Makeover television: Realities remodeled*. London: I.B. Taurus.

Kompridis, N. (2008). The unsettled and unsettling claims of culture: A reply to Seyla Benhabib. *Political Theory, 34*, 389–397. Retrieved from http://sagepub.com.

Leppert, A. & Wilson, J. (2008). Living the hills life: Lauren Conrad as reality star, soap opera heroine, and brand. *Genders, 48.* Retrieved from http://www.genders.org/g48/g48_leppertwilson.html

Miller, T. (2007). *Cultural citizenship: Cosmopolitanism, consumerism, and television in a neoliberal age.* Philadelphia: Temple UP.

Morley, D. (2000). *Home territories: Media, mobility and identity.* New York: Routledge.

Ouellette, L. (2009). Take responsibility for yourself: Judge Judy and the neoliberal citizen. In L. Ouellette & S. Murray (Eds.). *Reality TV: Remaking television culture.* (2nd ed.) (pp. 223–242). New York and London: NYU Press.

Redden, G. (2007). Makeover morality and consumer culture. In D. Heller (Ed.). *Makeover television: Realitie remodeled* (pp. 150–164). London: I.B. Taurus.

Sakai, N. (1997). *Translation and subjectivity: On "Japan" and cultural nationalism.* Minneapolis: UM Press.

5 Neoliberal Fantasies and the 'Centaur State': Confronting Hypermasculine Violence in Urban Public Schooling

Alexander J. Means

INTRODUCTION

This photo and quote from Oprah Winfrey (p. 98) represents a succinct crystallization of dominant ideology, or what Slavoj Žižek (1994), following Jacques Lacan, might refer to as the neoliberal 'fantasy.' This fantasy is based on the idea that 'society,' understood as a totality of integrated relationships, does not, in fact, exist; only impersonal market exchanges, private choices, and individual psyches. This fantasy, which Oprah's quote encapsulates, reveals the utopian dimension of neoliberal capitalism alongside its gendered logic. The subject of ideology here is, of course, a man, who is interpellated to reconstruct the future through the recalibration of 'his' consciousness. Not only are women and girls written out of this fantasy and therefore silenced, but so too are the everyday forms of insecurity and violence that mark our present historical moment, particularly in the lives of women. These deconstructive observations concerning ideology and silencing perhaps take on additional significance and meaning when one considers that I took this photograph inside a public high school located in an economically devastated and racially segregated neighborhood in Chicago. (Along with pseudonyms used for participants, I refer to this school as Carter High School [CHS] and the neighborhood as Ellison Square). A junior named Olivia describes Ellison Square and CHS in this way:

> When you go to this neighborhood you might see the signs in the yards that say "Bank of America failed this home and I lost it to foreclosure." Things like that affect people's mentalities. Again maybe if we were in a suburb where everything was nice and clean and it was low gang violence outside of school then maybe the inside of school would be a less violent place. . . . We just accept the fact that because we are all minorities and we live in this neighborhood that we're treated second rate. There are dirty rotten books and broken desks and graffiti everywhere. It just kind of adds to that. It's like you're looking for someone to blame and you can just go up the ladder but eventually you don't know who else to blame. You can blame your principal, but your principal has someone to blame because she's got a boss, and her boss's boss has a

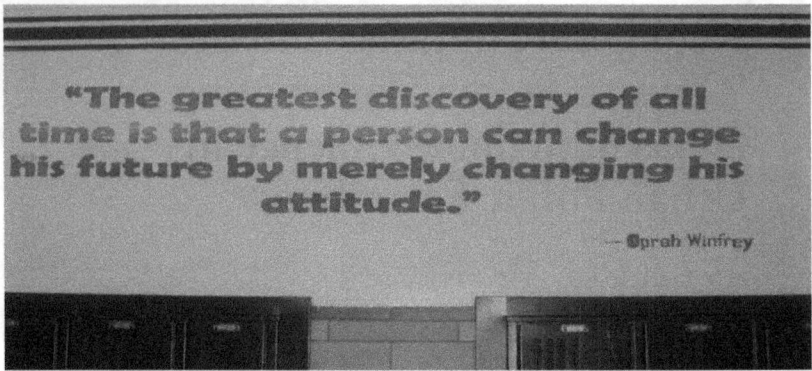

Figure 5.1   Author photograph from a hallway in Carter High School in Chicago.

boss. So I don't know. It's a hierarchy. You just have to climb the ladder and ask who is ultimately to blame.

Olivia's comments provide an interesting counterpoint to Oprah's fantasy. Rather than blame herself or her peers, Olivia observes that 'people's mentalities' are inextricably linked to broader economic conditions and political decisions that define relations of power and privilege across urban geographies. She also insightfully recognizes the connection between inequality and violence in her school and community. In my book, *Schooling in the Age of Austerity: Urban Education and the Struggle for Democratic Life* (2013), I examined the perspectives of youths like Olivia and teachers at CHS in order to shed light on the dynamics of urban and educational change.[1] I found that youths and adults at CHS held complicated and often conflicted views in relation to their school, neighborhood, and city, resisting as well as reproducing individual and psychological explanations for social instability, violence, and inequality. This chapter draws on this work in order to reflect specifically on the *androcentric violence* inherent to neoliberal urbanism and the restructuring of public schooling. Using the perspectives of teachers and youth as empirical anchoring points, I elaborate here how gendered transformations at the level of capital and the state are implicated in objective articulations of violence within urban educational policy, sociality, and everyday life. In conclusion, I build on Nancy Fraser's work to argue that urban educational studies require renewed focus on the relationship between gender and capitalism in an era of spiraling neoliberal crisis.

FROM A 'CRISIS OF MASCULINITY' TO SYSTEMIC GENDERED VIOLENCE

Urban violence is inextricably tied in the media to images of young men of color, guns, and street gangs. This association between violence and men has been understood in part through a pervasive 'crisis of masculinity' said to afflict poor urban communities. The crisis of masculinity suggests that men of color are inherently pathological. This takes concrete form in narratives of absent and irresponsible fathers, male sexual promiscuity, unruly boys failing in schools, male joblessness, and male criminality ('thugs' and 'gang bangers'). These representations typically circulate in historically and socially decontextualized ways, yet they have deep historical roots in racist stereotypes and forms of racist exploitation going back to slavery, reconstruction, and Jim Crow. The crisis of masculinity is also reflected in conservative social science discourse as well. Daniel Patrick Moynihan's (1966) influential analysis of the supposed cultural pathology of 'matriarchal' black families in the 1960s is a key social science touchstone. The crisis of masculinity and the focus on urban young men of color tend to overshadow the everyday struggles facing young women in their homes, on their streets, and in their schools. Maya, a sophomore at CHS, recalls a shooting that occurred on the front lawn of the school while she was in class:

> I was in my class. I was in my division. I was right there because we were looking through the window. It was hot so we had opened the windows and we were looking out the window and we just saw the boy had just got shot and he was just lying there and somebody was like, "Get help." And that's when the teacher told us to sit down. All I saw was a car pulled over and the boy was just walking and they shot him. And that's when the teacher was like, "Sit down, stop instigating" and stuff like that. . . . I just felt hurt.

Such horrific instances of gun violence and the trauma they inflict upon all those touched by them understandably elicit strong responses to make urban neighborhoods and schools safer and more secure. However, the way we make sense of such violence presents both limitations and possibilities for how we formulate our efforts to prevent violence and promote substantive forms of security. Slavoj Žižek (2008) offers a useful diagram in this regard. He suggests there are three interwoven types of violence:

1 Subjective: the violence perpetrated by individuals or 'identifiable agents;'
2 Symbolic: the violence embedded within language and aesthetic and cultural representation;
3 Systemic: the structural violence inhered within late modern societies.

For Žižek (2008), 'subjective' violence is only the most visible of the three. This privatized or individualized form of violence appears to us as a disruption to the 'normal' state of things, such as in school shootings or in spectacular acts of terrorism. In contrast, as 'objective' forms, systemic and symbolic violence refer to the violence inhered directly within this 'normal' state of things—within the "smooth functioning of our economic and political systems" (Žižek, 2008, p. 2). Whereas objective violence may be less visible than subjective forms, it is no less visceral or real in its effects. Žižek states that:

> systemic violence is thus like the "dark matter" of physics, the counterpart to an all-too visible subjective violence. It may be invisible, but it has to be taken into account if one is to make sense of what otherwise seem to be "irrational" explosions of subjective violence (p. 2).

Žižek's (2008) analysis suggests that rather than something exceptional, violence is, in fact, quite ordinary, embedded within the normal functioning of global capitalism and the neoliberal state. These insights are essential for broadening our view of violence and can be read as deeply indebted to the work of those like Hannah Arendt and Pierre Bourdieu who have examined violence as immanent to capitalist modernity and its institutional, symbolic, and political economies. I suggest in the next section that in order to move beyond a reductive 'crisis of masculinity' narrative and, thus, properly understand the dimensions of violence within urban schools and communities, which Maya's comments viscerally capture, we need to look at gendered transformations of capital and the state under neoliberal urbanism that perpetuate androcentric violence.

THE HYPERMASCULINIZATION OF CAPITAL AND THE STATE IN AN ERA OF NEOLIBERAL REPRESSION

As a number of prominent scholars such as Wendy Brown (2005), Zygmunt Bauman (2001), Henry Giroux (2012), and David Harvey (2005) have detailed, the 'neoliberal revolution' that began to sweep across societies in the early 1980s has contributed to the disintegration of the social democratic consensus that held sway in the aftermath of the Great Depression and World War II. Whereas there has been a great deal of scholarly reflection on neoliberalism as a form of policy (Ball, 2012), an ideology (Hall, 2011), a cultural project (Giroux, 2012), a mode of governmentality (Foucault, 2008), and a reassertion of ruling class politics (Harvey, 2005), these perspectives have not typically focused on the gendered dimensions of neoliberal development. In the simplest terms, neoliberalism represents the 'hypermasculinization of state governance' vis-à-vis the vast expansion of state power steered by the rationalities and interests of transnational capital. Pierre Bourdieu (1999) describes this as the simultaneous erosion of the state's 'feminine' 'left arm' or social functions, and the expansion of its paternalistic or 'masculine' 'right arm'—those state capacities concerned with security, punishment, and policing. The nominally social democratic Keynesian welfare state operated to regulate capitalism and provide a modicum of protection against its most destructive tendencies. Under neoliberalism, the market becomes the internal regulator of the state, reducing its role in social reproduction while expanding its capacity for paternalistic repression. The sociologist Loic Wacquant

(2009) suggests that this hypermasculinization of the state in the neoliberal era of market fundamentalism and punitive neoconservatism has produced a double-movement. On the one hand, it has led to profound *social insecurity for a broad majority of citizens* through the evisceration of social investment and privatization of the public sphere, attacks on workers' rights and wages, and the unprecedented redistribution of wealth and power to the top of the social class hierarchy. On the other hand, it has led to *a penal spiral of criminalization and mass incarceration directed most acutely at those racialized spaces and stigmatized populations made redundant in the low-wage post-industrial economy*. Wacquant (2009) thus refers to the United States as a "centaur state," which he describes as:

> a free market head mounted on an authoritarian body . . . that applies the doctrine of "laissez-faire" upstream, when it comes to social inequalities and the mechanisms that generate them (the free play of capital, deregulation of labor law and deregulation of employment, retraction or removal of collective protections), but turns out to be brutally paternalistic and punitive downstream, when it comes to coping with their consequences on a daily level (p. 43).

For Wacquant (2009), the neoliberal government of social insecurity is an explicitly *gendered project of post-social population management* stemming from the reorganization of work in an era of precarious, service-based wage-labor. Women, particularly immigrant women and women of color, are more likely to occupy positions at the bottom of the wage scale and informal work sector, and, along with their children, bear the brunt of the effects of poverty. Whereas women and children are overrepresented among the working poor, men are far more likely to face chronic unemployment coupled with higher rates of imprisonment. Wacquant argues that 'workfare,' directed predominantly at managing low-wage female labor, and 'prisonfare,' aimed at managing unemployed men, functionally emerge as dominant race and gender-coded class strategies for governing surplus populations in the neoliberal city. As we will see in the section below, these governmental dynamics are articulated in urban educational contexts in specific ways along the lines of class, race, and urban spatial politics.

SPECTERS OF VIOLENCE IN URBAN EDUCATIONAL POLICY, SOCIALITY, AND EVERYDAY LIFE

Neoliberal urbanism can be characterized as a general trend toward the 'rolling back' of social democratic policy regimes and the 'rolling out' (Peck & Tickel, 2002) of market-based governance, consisting of a number of 'distinct tendencies,' including the privatization of urban institutions and services, attacks on public workers and unions (and their earned benefits), extensive tax breaks and incentives for corporate development and investment, and the criminalization of the urban poor. As scholars like Pauline Lipman (2011) have noted, educational privatization and the integration of corporate-driven market logics and criminalizing practices into the fabric of urban education are a succinct representation of neoliberal urbanism. In this section, I bring in the voices of teachers and youth at CHS in order to discuss how the restructuring urban public schools reflect the 'hypermasculinization of neoliberal power' and how this serves to perpetuate the objective realities of androcentric violence in urban schools and communities.

Whereas Ellison Square is only a short distance from the glittering office towers, professional class jobs, tourist attractions, and trendy shops of downtown Chicago, it exists as a world set apart. Wacquant (2008) has described urban neighborhoods like Ellison Square and the sea of impoverished African American and Latino neighborhoods that border it on Chicago's Southside as twenty-first century hyperghettos: stigmatized zones of economic fragmentation and ethnoracial enclosure defined by the duel retrenchment in the labor market and social provision and the simultaneous extension of the surveillance and penal web of the neoliberal state. Ellison Square is marked by poverty and joblessness alongside limited access to stable employment opportunities, health care, transportation, and well-resourced schools. For many residents of Ellison Square, public disinvestment and budgetary crises have meant that access to social services comes in the form of a Mobile Community Center operated by the Department of Child and Family Services (DCFS). This is a bus that parks in the neighborhood once a month that serves as an all-in-one stand-in for what remains of the social arm of the state, offering limited access to job information, home foreclosure assistance, health and immunization services, and a food pantry. On the other end of the spectrum, there is an intensive and extensive security and law enforcement presence in the neighborhood. It is impossible not to notice the dozens of police surveillance cameras that blanket the area, hanging like strange mechanical fruit from telephone and light poles, expanding the gaze of law enforcement to virtually every intersection and sidewalk in the community. It is routine to witness police officers interrogating local youth on street corners or to see youth sprawled over the hoods or sitting handcuffed in the backseats of police cruisers. In these moments, the neighborhood has the feel of an occupied territory.

CHS and its grounds take up an entire city block in the middle of Ellison Square. The 80-year-old school serves a population of close to 2,000 students roughly split 50–50 between Latino and African American youth. These are high needs and high poverty students—90% of whom qualify for free or reduced lunch, 97% qualify as low-income, 18% are involved in special education, and 8% are English language learners. It is common to hear urban public schools like CHS described in the media and elsewhere as 'dumping grounds, schools of last resort, and as drop out factories.' These terms, of course, are pejorative and speak to the broad stigmatization of urban public schools as they are linked in the media to 'failure' and 'crisis.' Behind this rhetoric, however, lies a constellation of processes, policies, and political decisions that are eroding the human development capacities of public schools. Rooted in neoliberal ideologies that promise to ensure justice and equity through the supposed entrepreneurial efficiencies of markets and top-down corporate management, 150 public schools have been closed in Chicago over the last decade to make way for educational privatization and the creation of market-based school choice arrangements, charter schools, and selective enrollment schools.

Research has shown that selective enrollment and charter schools skim off students and funds from public schools like CHS (Catalyst, 2010). As these privatized schools are often able to selectively choose their students, and as school funding and contract renewals are increasingly linked to test scores under high stakes accountability measures, 'high performing' students become 'valued commodities' whereas 'low performing' students, students with learning disabilities and English language learners, are characterized as 'undesirables' and 'outcasts.' In the wake of public school closures and turn-arounds, the vast majority of students, who are typically the most academically and socially in need, are sent packing. According to the Consortium on School Research at the University of Chicago, only 6% of displaced students from school closures end up enrolling in academically 'strong' schools. The majority of displaced students, some 82%, re-enter other 'low performing' public schools such as CHS (Gwynne & de la Torre, 2009). As a result, and like its counterparts across the US, urban public schools like CHS are thus increasingly becoming 'warehouses' and 'containment centers' for students with the greatest needs and from the most disadvantaged backgrounds, and for whom English is a second language.

> (Ms. Douglas, teacher at CHS): The school has been set up by the system for failure. Basically, we have magnet schools that skim the more academically aggressive kids and the kids whose parents can find a better option so we're kind of known as a school of last resort. There is a set-up right there. Number two, we must take everybody who comes, so we get the kids that are kicked out of charter schools, we get the kids that are getting let out of jail and coming back from alternative schools, and we take everyone. At the same time, when you have selective enrollment schools skimming your most academic students and then you get the reputation of being a school of last resort, then there are some issues with the attitude people have toward the school and sadly a mindset on the part of the kids. . . . So we're set up for failure in that way. . . . The other way the system treats us is like a number. Every 400 kids, one security guard. Eighteen-hundred kid school and we are entitled to four security guards which is preposterous, so the school has to dip into its own discretionary funds and buy security guards with it. So instead of lowering class sizes, adding more teachers or resources, or any of those

choices that would help the kids, our school has to buy security guards in order to have a greater adult presence. . . . It would be great to have resources put into more social workers or psychologists that really could help the kids with some of the incredible issues that they bring to school, including anger over everything that they are dealing with. But instead those meager resources go into security personnel. So instead we get all the kids that are kicked out and a disproportionate amount of kids that are lower academically than the selective enrollment schools. We have a disproportionate share of Special Ed students and yet we are compared to these schools with different circumstances and labeled as a failing or struggling school. . . . The fact is that the system has set up schools like ours as targets and then wonders why when they close surrounding schools and those low performers come to the school, the scores remain low. It's just a vicious cycle and I just can't get the logic of turning over schools to private organizations when in fact the leadership of the city is supposed to be in charge of them. It makes no sense. They neglect these schools, under resource them, and then blame them and say, "The answer is to turn them over to outside groups." It makes no sense.

Alongside privatization, patterns of austerity and social disinvestment are having a profound influence in shaping life at CHS. As demonstrated by the 2008 financial crisis and subsequent Wall Street bailouts, neoliberal capitalism relies on a muscular state in order to ameliorate market failure and upwardly redistribute wealth and power, while downwardly distributing fiscal austerity, debt, and precariousness onto the public sphere and to communities. Students and teachers frequently spoke of how worsening poverty stemming from the great recession has generated myriad problems such as homelessness, mental health and addiction issues, and stability of home life. Here a teacher named Mr. Bradley pushes back against the neoliberal fantasy of individual and psychological roots of social insecurity and the discourse of meritocratic mobility:

Lots of kids have lost their place and have had parents who have lost their jobs and have been foreclosed on. There are students who are just simply homeless. This one girl in my AP class, her family is intact and they seem like a great family, but the father lost his job and then they lost the house and so now they have been living out of a car for a while. So homework becomes out of the question and her focus has shifted from school to finding a job in order to help her family. And she is not the only one. . . . And you know, you hear on like Oprah that inspiring story about the girl who overcomes that and goes to Harvard and that's awesome, but that girl is not like the rest of us. She is to be admired, but such things are not done even by the best of people, it's just too much to overcome.

Teachers and students often spoke to the objective connections between poverty, emotional trauma, and violence at CHS, and there is a broad feeling and recognition that the services available for students in the school and community are totally inadequate for addressing these concerns. For instance, CHS has only one social worker for its nearly 2,000 students, and the students are allotted a maximum of 15 minutes a month with her. The lack of support services for youth only underscores more generalized conditions of austerity. Many classrooms do not have enough desks, as budget cuts have swelled class sizes. It is common to see packed classrooms with students sprawled about, sitting on the edges of the class, and even some standing without desks. The class size issue underscores a more general absence of books and other essential resources. Teachers have routinely reached into their own pockets in order to cover the costs of basic supplies, such as photocopies of class textbooks due to their insufficient number. Further, the school not only has a shortage of supplies but a shortage of teachers as well. Over the summer of 2010, the school had to layoff approximately 15% of its faculty due to budget cuts in the aftermath of the 2008 economic crisis and recession. In the wake of the layoffs, the school is using what they call 'placeholders'—transient substitutes who are something like the educational equivalent of the service sector 'permatemp:' Ms. Lorrie, a science teacher, expresses her frustration at these conditions:

> I feel like the schools are looked at as this net that is placed below the community, but not just a net because we obviously have the primary focus of educating the kids and that will hopefully help get them out of poverty, but I feel like anything else that might impact our primary focus, we are expected to catch the community. Like, "Oh well, your kids can't focus because they are hungry so we'll have reduced breakfast and lunch and summer meal programs" and things like that. Like, "Your kids can't get access to health care so we'll have the immunization bus come out once a year because they have to have that to get into school." Like, "There was a shooting last night, so we'll bring in crisis counselors." But I feel like it's not even a safety net. I feel like it's just reactionary. I feel like the school is just scrambling, trying to figure out how to provide the bare minimum so that kids can potentially have a half of a prayer of getting out the door with an education.

The destabilizing effects of privatization and austerity are further extended in the realm of teaching and learning. Despite the efforts of teachers to provide meaningful and engaging lessons, there is a strong feeling among faculty that they are limited by an inflexible 'direct instructional' and 'scripted' curricular approach that emphasizes basic skills and standardized testing at the expense of creative learning. This curriculum, much of it developed and contracted out to educational corporations, is often of questionable relevance to students' lives and experiences. A teacher named Mr. Parks elaborates:

> There are four sets of clipboards that come through my classroom. Number one is IDS. But IDS is not aligned with RTI. RTI is not aligned with Area 23. And Area 23 which wants the skills and standards to be the Illinois State are not aligned with the College Readiness. So unless I know who you are coming into my classroom, I don't know how to sequence the skills that my kids need to be learning in order to meet the expectations placed on me to teach these ridiculous things. As their teacher, I've got a pretty good idea of which skills I need to start sequencing to get them to the level in which to function in today's society, but those four competing clipboards have no relevance. They're each connected to different money and different programs, each of which have a competing and conflicting interest in what happens in my classroom. The curriculum is not just the curriculum; it's a loaded political football from the Gates Foundation to IDS and Kaplan that's making an awful lot of money on what I'm teaching. And in this day and age, content is just not all that important. It's about the skills being taught and that's really not all that content based. . . . At the present time, every week we get something else added to our instructional clock, to our curriculum, and administrators have stopped even trying to justify their way. They've just been mandated; that's why we do it. And that's where children of poverty and children of such institutions continue to be raped by the educational system. It's because if you try to get away with mandating this at a middle class suburban school like Walter Paten or North Side High School you would be burned at the stake. Who in the hell gives you the right to do it to our school?

The emphasis on testing and basic skills in low-achieving and socially disinvested public schools reproduces broader conditions of masculinized structural violence and inequality where, through narrow and rudimentary curricula, most CHS students will be primarily sorted into spaces at the lowest end of the service based job market or will be pushed out of school and the formal economy altogether. Shahrzad Mojab and Sara Carpenter (2011) have described such socio-pedagogical relations as 'learning by dispossession,' whereby young people are disconnected from the forms of learning and knowledge necessary to understand, overcome, and transform the conditions in which they live. It is in this context of austerity and dispossession that the 'right arm' of hypermasculinized state violence and criminalization of educational environments must be understood. CHS represents a militarized space where youth are routinely subject to harsh forms of surveillance and discipline. When entering the school, one is greeted by uniformed security guards, armed police, airport style x-ray screeners, scanning wands, and metal detectors. Inside the school, metal cages on the windows, steel cages over doors, cages that can be expanded across hallways during 'lockdowns,' ubiquitous surveillance cameras, and dim fluorescent-lit hallways all conjure prison aesthetics. At CHS, youth are routinely suspended, expelled, threatened with arrest, or arrested for what are often trivial offenses like 'talking back' to security guards and staff. A student named Olivia here describes this culture of punishment and repression:

> It's very reminiscent of a prison. Even though I've never been in prison, but it is reminiscent. Like, "Why are we treated like this?" I haven't done anything bad but I kind of have to pay by having to be searched by the metal detectors or having to be caught in a hall sweep. It does make you feel—if you treat me like a dog I might want to react like a dog. It does explain why some of the students act the way they do. Like I said, it's bad energy that you're giving, and I'm gonna give it right back. That's just how people are. But the thing is you kind of learn to just take what you're given. We don't think about these things. When you're walking down the hallway, it just kind of blends in to your everyday—it's like your mentality. You're like, "just take it" because it's where you are from and a lot of times you think it's just not gonna get any better. I mean, if you strive for better, you'll get better but a lot of people are like, "Well, if you can maintain then you can do it." This is not necessarily what I want for the rest of my life. I don't want to have to deal with just watching people fall. I don't think anyone should want that.

REFRAMING VIOLENCE THROUGH RADICAL FEMINIST CRITIQUE

The hypermasculinization of urban governance under neoliberalism produces new circulations of systemic inequality and gendered violence. These dynamics are all too visible within the city of Chicago and its disinvested working-class African American and Latino neighborhoods and public schools such as Ellison Square and CHS. Rather than investing in public education, job training, health care, restorative justice, and other measures that could work to reduce structural androcentric violence and, therefore, support a more robust notion of human security and democracy in urban neighborhoods and schools, cities like Chicago have embraced free market policies that erode public education and produce extreme inequality. At the same time, billions of dollars are poured into hypermasculinized law enforcement measures. These repressive security and containment strategies, such as ubiquitous surveillance cameras and zero-tolerance policing, may provide a veneer of safety against the very real threat of gun violence in and around poverty-stricken schools like CHS, but they do nothing to address the root causes and insecurities driving such violence in urban neighborhoods and schools.

In their book, *The Spirit Level*, epidemiologists Richard Wilkinson and Kate Pickett (2009) present a transnational comparative study of sociological data that unequivocally concludes,

> the association between inequality and violence is strong and consistent; it's been demonstrated in many different time periods and settings. Recent evidence of the close correlation between ups and downs in inequality and violence show that if inequality is lessened, levels of violence also decline (p. 144).

Wilkinson and Pickett indicate that the linkage between inequality and violence is multidimensional, involving struggles over access to economic and social resources as well as over cultural capital and social status. However, in their trenchant analysis of the transnational data, they find the social factors that contribute to high levels of subjective violence, such as low educational attainment, family breakdown, high levels of stress and depression, drug and alcohol abuse, and social mistrust, all correlate to the relative distribution of income, power, and wealth in a society. In short, what matters is not how affluent a society is but how unequal it is; that is, the more unequal the society, the more socially atomized and objectively and subjectively violent it becomes. Importantly, young men and women experience the hypermasculinized character of neoliberal violence and inequality differently. For instance, young men I spoke with in Ellison Square reported they are more likely to experience harassment and brutality by police. The following is a dialogue between a young man, Darien, and me:

ALEX: What's the relationship like between the police and students in the neighborhood?
DARIEN: I think the relationship is that the police, when they see people outside sometimes—it depends on who it is—but sometimes the cops, they're around and trying to figure things out and catch what's going on, but sometimes the police officer there will let you go if you give them information. Sometimes they come up to you for no reason and try to get information out of you.
ALEX: What kind of information?
DARIEN: Information like, "Do you know this person?" or "Where this person be?" or "What did they do at this person's house?" and things like that. Sometimes the police officers—there are racist police officers around here. Like, a couple of months ago a detective car, they grabbed this one guy like they were gonna arrest him and put him in the back of the car and took him somewhere and they beat

him up, and then they put him back in the car and dropped him back off and things like that just for no reason.

ALEX: Has this kind of thing happened to you?

DARIEN: It happens to me all the time. I'll be outside and they'll stop me and pat me down and ask me questions. . . . Like, one time they stopped us we were just walking down the street and this was before curfew, so we were just walking down the street, and this cop pulled over and pulled their guns on us and pushed us against the car. That was unnecessary. We wouldn't have resisted. When they pulled up next to us we stopped, we didn't keep going we stopped, and I just think all of that is unnecessary.

Whereas young women are exposed to these same conditions of repression, they are more likely to cite sexual violence and harassment as their primary concerns. McCormick (2003) found in her study of youth in an urban school in New York that female students experience the 'twin abuses' of both racism and sexism in their everyday lives at school and in their communities. McCormick observed that female students often have to develop strategies to 'shield' themselves from unwanted sexual attention, harassment, and intimidation on the streets and in their schools. A student named Sasha elaborates:

As a female I've been checked by a lot of grown men and that's what I've gotta worry about. For example, me and my cousin we used to go to the store outside and people would stop their cars and try to talk to me and stuff like that. And I try to avoid that because my dad is really overprotective of me because I'm an only child and my mother passed away so he's really protective of me. And if he ever sees something like that he's gonna go crazy. That's why I try to prevent everything from happening.

These specific gendered articulations of violence inherent to a hypermasculinized neoliberal state need to be further studied and documented by researchers in relation to the transformation of urban geographies and public institutions like urban public schools. Importantly, I believe this task requires reengagement with what Nancy Fraser (2013) has referred to as feminism's 'insurrectionary spirit,' which, she argues, reached its zenith during the second wave movements in the post-war era. As Fraser documents, second wave feminists sought to radicalize the social democratic imaginary that held sway in the aftermath of World War II that assumed class redistribution as a baseline for securing cross-class solidarity. Many attempted to do so by beginning to "question core features of capitalist modernity that social democracy had hitherto naturalized: materialism, consumerism, and the 'achievement ethic;' bureaucracy, corporate culture, and 'social control;' sexual repression, sexism, and heteronormativity" (Fraser, 2013, p. 3). As such, many second wave feminists crucially sought to expand social critique beyond an emphasis on class and redistributive politics into the arena of cultural recognition (e.g., civil rights and formal equality in law, employment, sexual relations, and language). Fraser argues that this project sought to deepen the socialist possibilities inherent to social democracy by expanding conceptions of social and gender justice through a sustained critique of institutional and cultural exclusions. Importantly, as Fraser recognizes, this turn to cultural recognition was strongly influenced by an emerging criticism of the white, western, and class privileged focus of the second wave movement itself, which was articulated by feminists of color and feminists from the global South (Chrenshaw, 1989; Collins, 1990, 2008; Mohanty, 1991; Spivak, 2005).

The neoliberal evisceration of social democracy beginning in the 1980s coincided with the retreat of feminist critique of capitalist society and its inherent androcentrism(s). What emerged in its place was a watered-down postmodern feminism, which, according to Fraser (2013), "often took the form of identity politics, aimed more at valorizing cultural difference than at promoting economic equality" (p. 4). Lost in this post-socialist feminist zeitgeist was the deeper structural analysis of capitalism and its moral and political economies of domination and exploitation that second wave feminism assumed as a baseline to cultural struggle. The profound global crisis of neoliberalism is wreaking havoc on the lives of working people and women across communities. As Fraser contends, this demands a reinvigoration of struggles over redistribution and recognition through a reflective, collaborative, and explicit feminist analysis of capitalism and its state forms. The brief ethnographic discussion I have offered in this chapter is an attempt to conduct such a feminist structural analysis of urban schooling that moves beyond the reductive neoliberal fantasy of individual and psychological explanations of violence and social inequality. As contributors to this volume argue, we need more focused scholarship and activism that confronts how contemporary androcentric power relations are functioning to limit the freedom and life of men and women throughout society through various modes of public repression, such as through the privatization and militarization of urban public schools. This work needs to be connected to ethical projects and movements aimed at dismantling the hypermasculine violence inherent to neoliberal policies, ideologies, and class/race/gender arrangements. This requires not only reviving a sense of radical democracy, but efforts to deepen and radicalize its solidaristic and egalitarian impulses in order to create more just, sustainable, non-alienated, and non-violent futures for all.

NOTE

1   I spent one semester doing ethnographic observations in and around Ellison Square and CHS and conducted 25 formal interviews and dozens of informal interviews with students, teachers, youth workers, police, security guards, parents, and staff. For more on my methods see (Means, 2013).

REFERENCES

Ball, S. (2012). *Global education inc: New policy networks and the neoliberal imaginary.* New York: Routledge.

Bauman, Z. (2001). *The individualized society.* New York: Polity.

Bourdieu, P. (1999). *Acts of resistance: Against the tyranny of the market.* New York, NY: New Press.

Brown, W. (2005). *Edgework: Critical essays on knowledge and politics.* Princeton, NJ: Princeton University Press.

Catalyst. (2010). Renaissance 2010. *Catalyst,* xxi(4). Retrieved from http://www.catalystchicago.org/sites/catalyst-chicago.org/files/assets/20100803/catsummer2010.pdf

Chrenshaw, K. (1989). *Demarginalizing the intersection of race and sex: A Black feminist critique of antidiscrimination doctrine, feminist theory and antiracist politics.* Chicago: University of Chicago Legal Forum, 139–167.

Collins, P. (1990/2008). *Black feminist thought.* New York: Routledge.

Foucault, M. (2008). *The birth of biopolitics: Lectures at the Collège de France, 1978–79.* New York: Palgrave Macmillan.

Fraser, N. (2013). *Fortunes of feminism: From state-managed capitalism to neoliberal crisis.* New York: Verso.

Giroux, H. (2012). *Twilight of the social: Resurgent publics in the age of disposability.* Boulder, CO: Paradigm.

Gwynne, J., & de la Torre, M. (2009). When schools close: Effects on displaced students in Chicago Public Schools. Consortium on Chicago School Research, University of Chicago. Retrieved from http://ccsr.uchicago.edu/content/publications.php?pub_id=136

Hall, S. (2011). *The neoliberal revolution: Thatcher, Blair, Cameron—the long march of neoliberalism continues.* Retrieved from http://www.lwbooks.co.uk/register.php?r=ReadingRoom/Hall.pdf

Harvey, D. (1991). *The condition of postmodernity.* New York: Wiley-Blackwell.

Harvey, D. (2005). *A brief history of neoliberalism.* Oxford, UK: Oxford University Press.

Lipman, P. (2011). *The new political economy of urban education: Neoliberalism, race, and the right to the city.* New York: Routledge.

McComick, J. (2003). Drag me to the asylum: Disguising and asserting identities in an urban school. *The Urban Review, 35*(2), 111–128.

Means, A. J. (2013). *Schooling in the age of austerity: Urban education and the struggle for democratic life.* New York: Palgrave Macmillan.

Mohanty, C. (1991). Under Western eyes: Feminist scholarship and colonial discourses. In C. Mohanty, A. Russo, & L. Torres (Eds.), *Third World women and the politics of feminism* (pp. 51–80). Bloomington, IN: Indiana University Press.

Mojab, S., & Carpenter, S. (2011). Learning by dispossession: Democracy promotion and civic engagement in Iraq and the United States. *International Journal of Lifelong Learning, 30*(4), 549–563.

Moynihan, D. P., Rainwater, L., &Yancey, W. L. (1966). *The Negro family: The case for national action.* Washington, DC: Office of Planning and Research, United States Department of Labor.

Peck, J., & Tickel, A. (2002). Neoliberalizing space. In N. Brenner & N. Theodore (Eds.), *Spaces of neoliberalism: Urban restructuring in North America and Western Europe.* Oxford, UK: Blackwell.

Spivak, G. C. (2005). *In other worlds: Essays on cultural politics.* New York: Routledge.

Wacquant, L. (2008). *Urban outcasts: A comparative sociology of advanced marginality*. Malden, MA: Polity.
Wacquant, L. (2009). *Punishing the poor: The neoliberal government of social insecurity*. Durham, NC: Duke University Press.
Wilkinson, R., & Pickett, K. (2009). *The spirit level: Why greater equality makes societies stronger*. New York: Bloomsbury Press.
Žižek, S. (1994). *The metases of enjoyment*. New York: Verso.
Žižek, S. (2008). *Violence*. New York: Picador.

6 'Prisonization' and Latinas in Alternative High Schools

Aida Hurtado, Ruby Hernandez, and Craig Haney

A recent *Huffington Post* exposé, "Prisoners of Profit," revealed extensive mistreatment of youth in "for profit" juvenile institutions caused by undertrained staff. The young women confined in these institutions were subjected to humiliating treatment and deprived of basic necessities (such as tampons and toilet paper). Unfortunately, the mistreatment of young, "at risk" women is not restricted to juvenile detention centers but also occurs, albeit in different ways, in many alternative educational settings. Long before they arrive at highly restrictive juvenile justice institutions, many young boys *and* girls have already attended other highly exclusionary institutions—so-called "alternative high schools."

Alternative high schools are supposedly designed for students who do not "fit" within "one size fits all" mainstream schools that cannot adequately address their unique educational and emotional needs. They are diverted to alternative high schools especially when this lack of fit contributes to increased levels of truancy, substance abuse, and disruptive behaviors like verbal conflicts and even fighting. A number of commentators have observed that even traditional public high schools have social psychological features that parallel those that exist in correctional institutions such as jails and prisons (e.g., Haney & Zimbardo, 1973). But we believe there are additional aspects of at least some alternative high schools that make the parallels even clearer and intensify the potentially negative consequences for the students who attend them.

The fact that young boys predominate in these places may help to explain why the "gendered educational pipeline" is so poorly understood or addressed in academic literature (Hurtado & Sinha, in press). Although alternative high schools are predominantly populated by youth of color, especially young men (Malagon, 2010; Malagon & Alvarez, 2010), increasingly there are more young Latinas in these institutions. Their considerably lower numbers perhaps account for the relative lack of direct analyses of how and why their experiences and needs differ from those of young men in general, and young Latinos in particular. In this chapter, we investigate specific vulnerabilities young Latinas experience (high levels of sexism, exposure to violence, and derailment from attending higher education beyond high school) created by larger social and institutional structures designed for young men. Taking an intersectional theoretical lens, we hope to avoid making young Latinas invisible by taking into account how their lives are experienced at the intersections of sexuality, gender, race, class, and ethnicity.

Many young Latinas are first generation in this country and many come from families not familiar with the US educational system at the high school level. Without full knowledge of the consequences, they accede to placement in alternative high schools where, in many cases, they are further marginalized. Some experience extreme forms of mistreatment, including psychological and even physical violence. Our ethnographic study focuses on some of their experiences in the course of this potentially marginalizing and psychologically traumatizing trajectory. We begin by providing a brief overview of alternative high schools in the United States.

OVERVIEW OF ALTERNATIVE HIGH SCHOOLS

The rise of "alternative schools" began in the late 1950s and early 1960s, when the Civil Rights Movement focused heightened public and political attention on the inequality and racism of traditional public education (Lange and Sletten, 2002). Raywid (1981) described these traditional public schools as "cold, dehumanizing, irrelevant institutions, largely indifferent to the humanity and the 'personhood' of those within them" (p. 551). According to Lange and Sletten (2002),

> At the same time, America was declaring a war on poverty, and in the Elementary and Secondary Education Act of 1965, President Johnson named the public school system as the front line of attack. . . . With government backing and funding, a new wave of alternatives was spawned that was meant to offer equal and meaningful education to disadvantaged and minority students (p. 3).

Although many of the programs and schools that arose from that era failed to achieve their stated goals, the legacy of this movement was the acknowledgement that not all students could succeed in mainstream high schools, underscoring a need for alternatives to accommodate different types of students. However, critical commentary about the potential drawbacks of these alternative school placements surfaced as early as the 1970s. Critics noted that the concentration of "at-risk" students (commonly referred to as "disadvantaged" and "disruptive" students), who were given little or no choice in whether to attend these schools, led to a series of presumably unintended consequences that compromised their educational mission and worsened many of the very problems they were intended to address (Carver, Lewis, & Tice, 2010; Lange & Sletten, 2002, p. 9). Of course, neither these criticisms nor the ones we advance in this chapter apply to all such schools, nor are they intended to stigmatize the staff who work in them or the students who attend. Rather, our goal is to draw attention to a presumably well-intentioned reform that in many instances not only fails to achieve its stated purpose, but also does so in a way that differentially affects students of color.

The current definition of what constitutes an "alternative high school" is difficult to specify. Federal-level definitions vary from state-level definitions as well as from state to state (and, at times, even within states) (Lange & Sletten, 2002; Lehr, Tan, & Ysseldyke, 2000). Alternative high schools tend to go by many names, including "continuation high schools," "alternative high schools," and "transfer high schools." They share the common purpose of educating "at-risk" students who either have opted out of the mainstream high school system or were deemed by school authorities to be unsuited for mainstream schooling. Although some "alternative" high schools are designed to provide especially innovative forms of education, few students who have social, economic, and educational vulnerabilities attend them. For the purpose of this chapter, we use "alternative high schools" to indicate high schools as described by Carver et al. (2010):

> Alternative schools and programs are designed to address the needs of students that typically cannot be met in regular schools. The students who attend alternative schools and programs are typically at risk of educational failure, as indicated by poor grades, truancy, disruptive behavior, pregnancy, or similar factors associated with temporary or permanent withdrawal from school. (p. 1)

Students who attend these schools are considered to be temporarily or permanently withdrawn or excluded from mainstream schools. They include students who are homeless, have formerly dropped out of school, and are children of migrant workers (Gable, Bullock, & Evans, 2006; Parsons, 2013) as well as English Language Learner (ELL) students (Lange & Sletten, 2002; Malagon & Alvarez, 2010), and students with disabilities ("Alternative Education About," 2008); Lehr et al., 2009).

THE GENDERED PIPELINE

The plight of young Latino men in the educational system is an important topic that approximately has been examined in the literature (e.g., Saenz & Ponjuan, 2009), along with the issue of specific gendered vulnerabilities (Hurtado & Sinha, in press). In this chapter, we acknowledge that there are important commonalities between young Latinos and Latinas that affect their school experiences. For example, both groups are likely to attend poor schools, represent the first generation to enter higher education, be raised in poverty, share immigrant status, and so on. Yet, despite these common structural positions, each group manifests the effects of their structural disadvantages in very different ways. In addition, they have experienced sometimes subtle but important differences in life experiences and gender socialization histories that help to account for their different levels of overall educational achievement (Hurtado, Haney, & Hurtado, 2012).

Thus, we contend that existing ethnic and racial group gender differences in educational experiences must be understood in the context of severe and persistent structural inequalities. Among Latinos/as, differences in educational achievement between girls and boys—including girls' higher rates of high school completion and college graduation—clearly do exist throughout the educational pipeline, as they do for African Americans at an even more disproportionate level (Saenz & Ponjuan, 2009). Some of these differences may be explained by recent historical developments and the different life experiences those events produced for young Latinos and Latinas. Most importantly, perhaps the feminist revolution that occurred over the last several decades sought and achieved greater educational equity for girls in general. Yet many of the gender equity programs that were designed largely for white women brought about positive change for Latinas as well (Corbett, Hill, & St. Rose, 2008). Because white men did not need a social and legal movement to enhance their already structurally privileged position, no comparable movement arose over the same time period from which Latino men could benefit.

Nonetheless, there are increasing numbers of young Latinas entering both alternative high schools and the criminal justice system. We believe that there are gender specific experiences and vulnerabilities that help to account for their presence in both of these settings. We examine these issues using the emerging literature on gender intersectional vulnerabilities in schooling and using examples from ethnographic data gathered in the context of one particular alternative high school in Northern California.

SITE DESCRIPTION

The Grove Continuation High School (GCHS) is situated in a moderately sized tourist city located in the Bay Area of California[1]. Although the town is mostly white (58.6 %), with a higher percentage of whites than in the state overall (39%), there is a sizeable Latino (32.9%) population as well (County QuickFacts from the US Census Bureau, 2014). During the 2011–12 school year, GCHS reported an enrollment of 111 high school students, with twice as many male students (68%) as female (32%) (California Department of Education, 2014). Fifty-nine percent of the students were Latino/a (35% Latinos, 24.3% Latinas), 31% were white (25.2% males, 5.4% females), 2.6% were Asian males (no females), 3% were African American males (no females), and 1.8% were mixed raced (1% female) or Native American (1% female). The latest enrollment figures indicate the Latina/o student population in GCHS is increasing, whereas the white student population is decreasing (the number of other students has remained basically the same).

The main reason that students are directed to alternative high schools (including GCHS) in the state is because they lack sufficient credits for graduation (Accrediting Commission for Schools, Western Association of Schools and Colleges [ASC WASC], 2009). Their lack of sufficient academic progress could have occurred for many reasons, including

> learning challenges, being a second language learner, irregular atten-
> dance and/or truancy, inappropriate behavior [such as disruptive behav-
> ior in class], family difficulties, job responsibilities [such as holding a
> job while in school and needing scheduling flexibility], child abuse/
> neglect, substance abuse, and teen pregnancy. (ASC WASC, 2009, p. 3)

Of the students at GCHS, fully 41% were English Language Learners (ELL), 69% were considered socioeconomically disadvantaged, and 7% were reported as having disabilities of some kind.

Of the eight GCHS faculty at the time of the study, seven identified as white (one chose not to identify his/her ethnicity and race). There were two who reported English/Spanish bilingual skills (ASC WASC, 2009). At least two of the faculty had previous experience working in alternative high schools. The number of white faculty was thus higher than the 67% state average of white teachers in California (California Department of Education, 2013). GCHS also employed part time support staff shared with other surrounding schools. Among these were counselors, school community coordinators, campus supervisors, health clerks, clerical specialists, food service workers, registrars, custodians, and the principal's secretary. At least six of the support staff were Spanish/English speakers (ASC WASC, 2009).

The ethnographic observations took place primarily in one class-room and occasionally in different parts of the high school. In addition, one semi-structured interview was conducted with the English teacher whose classroom was under observation. The interview was recorded and tran-scribed and, following standard procedures in ethnography, the field notes were also written up and analyzed (Emerson, Fretz, & Shaw, 2011; Fet-terman, 2010; Fine & Weis, 1998; Lofland & Lofland, 1995; Valenzuela, 1999). Many informal interviews were also conducted through conversa-tions with students, staff, and teachers during the ethnographic observa-tions. Field notes were generated during the breaks between class periods shortly after each class observation to ensure greater accuracy in recording the events. Most observations were recorded at the end of the day or within 24 hours after the observations. The ethnography was designed from within an intersectional theoretical framework. As noted below, this framework allowed us to take various axes of difference explicitly into account as we sought to understand how Latina students at GCHS experienced vulnera-bilities and potential violence at a predominantly male school environment.

INTERSECTIONAL CONSIDERATIONS

From the theoretical perspective of "intersectionality," there are certain dimensions or "axes" of difference in society that have special political, social, and economic implications. These axes traditionally include the social categorizations of race, class, sexuality, gender, and ethnicity (Collins, 2002; Hurtado, 1996). These particular social identities are part of the process of social categorization that is used by core institutions in our society to allocate power and privilege. As such, these categorizations and the social identities they produce have enormous consequences for the members of the groups to whom they are applied. Therefore, special attention has to be paid to well-defined samples that allow the desegregation of research results along these axes of difference.

We see intersectionality as an especially fruitful approach to the study of young Latinas (Hurtado, 2003; Hurtado, 2010; Hurtado & Cervantez, 2009). In this chapter, we use an intersectional approach to understand young Latinas attending alternative schools as they confront and negotiate the consequences and implications of class, sexuality, ethnicity, and race (phenotype) differences. As Hurtado and her colleagues found in their intersectional analysis of young Latinas in higher education, the participants' views on gender relations were directly affected by the participants' social class, phenotype (fair skinned versus dark skinned), and sexual orientation (Hurtado, 2003; Hurtado, 2010; Hurtado & Cervantez, 2009). For example, Hurtado (2003) found Latinas of Mexican descent who had participated in education beyond high school through exposure to different classes in higher education were able to articulate the prior knowledge of the consequences of their phenotype—whether they were fair or dark skinned and whether their features were Anglo or indigenous (or African)-looking. The participants experienced racialization both within their families and in society.

Sexuality is also an important issue in understanding the full range of educational obstacles young Latinas may face. Although only three of 101 participants in Hurtado's (2003) study stated they were lesbian, and three were bisexual (or had relationships with women), these participants reported a number of distinctly different views and experiences as compared to the larger group. For example, almost all parents, other family members, and their communities did not necessarily accept their sexual orientation, although all of the respondents remained connected to their families (Hurtado, 2003).

GENDERED REACTIONS TO HYPER-MONITORING

Placing youth in alternative high schools is a potentially life altering experience that can have socially stigmatizing and structurally marginalizing consequences that undermine a person's chances for educational and occupational success. We argue below that these "alternative" educational institutions have a number of features in common with juvenile justice or correctional institutions and present students with many of the same kinds of psychologically powerful and potentially damaging experiences. Although sometimes subtle and not often explicitly "named," these experiences can have profound consequences for the life trajectory of students. As Haney (2003) has suggested, although much of the research on the negative consequences of incarceration has focused on "the most extreme or clinically diagnosable effects of imprisonment," there are "broader and subtler psychological changes that occur in the routine course of adapting to prison life" (p. 38).

Specifically, the process of institutionalization—called "prisonization" when it occurs in correctional settings—is the shorthand expression for

> a unique set of psychological adaptations that typically occur—in varying degrees—in response to the extraordinary demands of prison. In general terms, the process of prisonization involves the incorporation of the norms of prison life into one's habits of thinking, feeling, and acting. (Haney, 2003, p. 38)

Inmates reacting in psychologically limiting ways that impair their adjustment to normal relationships once they leave prison demonstrate prisonization. As proposed by Haney, prisonization entails six characteristics: 1) dependence on institutional structures and contingencies; 2) hyper-vigilance, interpersonal distrust, and suspicion; 3) overt emotional regulation, alienation, and psychological distancing; 4) social withdrawal and isolation; 5) incorporation of exploitive norms of prison culture; and 6) diminished sense of self-worth and personal value.

Procedures and practices within many alternative high schools implement prison-like hyper-monitoring that is directed at students and justified on the basis of assumptions made about their alleged histories of past misbehavior. At GCHS, the students were closely monitored through a system that awarded "credits" for participation and attendance. Students also were systematically disciplined for undesirable behaviors such as tardiness and failing to complete their assignments. The system of rewards and punishments was quite elaborate. Students sardonically referred to one salient mechanism of control as "The Box"—the disciplinary detention room where they were sent when other sanctions failed to produce the desired effect. For example, a tardy student was sanctioned by being retained in "The Box" for double the amount of time he or she was late (e.g., a half hour punishment for being tardy by 15 minutes). However, according to school policy, the students could not be detained before or after school. Thus, assignment to "The Box" had to occur during school hours, paradoxically disrupting learning and potentially impacting graduation. The irony of the use of "The

Box" is its counterpart in prison where inmates are disciplined by being sent to "The Hole."

In fact, Hurtado et al. (2012) make the connection between disciplining norms in inner city high schools and the development of a "carceral consciousness" where the criminality of young people of color is assumed and innocence has to be proved:

> Youth of Color are not only more likely to be categorized as deviant others through the lens of this carceral consciousness but also to be seen by the larger society as deserving of criminal justice-like sanctions. They are also more likely to be policed by the state, which is poised to intervene at the slightest indication of criminal behavior—sometimes turning the presumption of innocence on its head, so that criminality is often assumed and it is innocence that must be demonstrated or proved—including inside increasingly "prisonized" inner city public schools where "zero tolerance" policies criminalize their behavior and newly installed security hardware and procedures subject them "to scrutiny by armed police, dogs, or metal detectors." (Hirschield, 2008, p. 80) In these ways, the emerging carceral mentality produces a seamless continuation of the norms and dynamics of prison life into communities of color themselves. (p. 110)

The hyper-monitoring experienced by students at GCHS was reminiscent of total institutions like juvenile hall and in many ways the antithesis of what psychologists have called "self-efficacy." As Bandura (1995) defines it, self-efficacy is "the belief in one's capabilities to organize and execute the courses of action required to manage prospective situations" (p. 2). Persons who are high in self-efficacy believe in their ability to succeed in many different situations and, perhaps not surprisingly, this belief is significantly related to success and achievement in a range of settings. The hyper-monitoring encoded in numerous rules characteristic of alternative high schools undermines self-efficacy by teaching students to relinquish control to more powerful (and seemingly arbitrary) forces, to do so unquestioningly, and with respect to nearly every decision one might make on a daily basis.

In significant ways, the students at GCHS were being coerced into doing their schoolwork rather than internalizing an achievement motivation to become academically engaged. In fact, in extreme cases, hyper-monitoring enforced in alternative high schools such as GCHS may not only suppress self-efficacy but even push students close to a state of "learned helplessness" (Seligman, 1975). In such situations, they may be unable to engage in affirmative decision-making and action initiation on their own. These youth may avoid situations where these things are called for because they experience them as painful and anxiety provoking. These behaviors are more likely to have life-altering consequences for Latina/o students, whose structural positioning makes them more vulnerable to substandard, prisonizing forms of education. The effects of being exposed to institutional hyper-monitoring are not gender or culturally neutral. Young Latinos and Latinas may take different adaptations to the process of institutional hyper-monitoring and their reactions to these experiences are often gendered in nature. For young Latino men, the loss of self-efficacy may lead to a form of reactance in which they are more likely to strike out against authority. It may impair their ability to distinguish authority figures' reasonable requests for restraint and compliance from authoritarian, absolutist, or abusive demands. Although these experiences may also provoke this kind of response in some young Latina women, many of them tend to quietly over-comply as a way to negotiate hyper-monitoring. In other words, they tend to become invisible. We found this was especially true at GCHS where they were a distinct numerical minority.

There are other gendered differences to the behavior of Latino students in these environments. For example, Valenzuela (1990) has reported that young Chicanas in high school acted as a strategic bridge between school authorities like teachers and principals to advocate on behalf of their "guys"—usually boyfriends, male friends, and male relatives. In addition, they would "supervise" the comings and goings of "their guys" and encourage them to comply with school rules. In contrast, young Chicano men were erratic in their school attendance and could not focus enough to accomplish the minimum requirements to survive in high school. Instead, many young Chicanos hid behind the type of hypermasculine pose of dismissive detachment and emotional distancing that is so functional in total institutions like juvenile hall and prison, but which obviates any real engagement or investment in their schoolwork. Ironically, many young Latinas can advocate for the men in their lives but are unable fully to enact their self-efficacy on their own behalf.

The emotional work that many young Latinas take on was evident in the following interaction at GCHS related in field notes. Carlos, a Latino student, "ditched" school and returned intoxicated to the classroom. He was interacting with his fellow Latina student, Carina, and the ethnographer:

> Carlos has his fists on his cheek, his elbows on his desk propping his head up.
> "Why are your eyes red?" Carina asks Carlos in a semi-teasing tone of voice.
> "They're not red. I'm just tired."
> "See," says Carina [addressing the ethnographer] and pulls, somewhat harshly, at one of his fists revealing his very pink cheeks. I [the ethnographer] thought it was because he had his fists on his face.
> Carina continues in a semi-accusing tone asking Carlos. "How many did you have?"
> He replies, "One."
> Carina responds in a skeptical tone, "One did that to you?"

"No, you don't know how many I had." The red in his cheeks indicates Carlos is probably drunk. Carina asks him where he got drunk and he explains he and his friends went to a park and drank Coronas [beer] during second period.

I asked him if the park was far and he says "No." I ask how he made it there and back and he says "*Cars*" in a condescending tone and gives me a look as if saying this was perfectly obvious. I say "Okay." I didn't know he had a car. Carina tells him to layoff. Carlos is telling Carina they [he and his friends] know someone who is over 21. She says she knows whom he is talking about. He tells her not to say who it is, probably so I cannot find out.

I want him to do his work and encourage him to look at his assignment. Carlos ignores me and instead he starts making fun of Lee [another student] who is not in class.

Carlos's behavior was not unusual. Students at GCHS were often late to class and rarely fully committed to their schoolwork, performing at a minimum level. Students said they felt the assignments were either out of the range of their academic skills or they thought the work was too simplistic and beneath them. Moreover, even when they were in attendance, they were not necessarily present with a "clear mind" because of drugs, alcohol, and emotional, social, and economic vulnerabilities.

In the above interaction, Carlos did not acknowledge Carina's concern and care even though it was expressed in a culturally specific form of mild chastising, as a kind of good natured teasing. Instead, her attention, however sardonically delivered, was expected and became the invisible emotional work performed by many young Latinas in school settings. Carina was not only trying to get Carlos to recognize his transgressions of "ditching," "drinking," and "driving while intoxicated," she was also trying to engage the ethnographer, perhaps at some level hoping that the ethnographer would "snitch" on Carlos and get him back on track. When the transgressions that sent the Latino boys to alternative schools were more severe, the Latina students were burdened with more significant emotional and psychological work. The effects of gender socialization seemed clear. There were no instances in which the gender roles were reversed and young Latinos provided emotional support, even in a teasing way, to Latina students.

Hyper-monitoring in alternative schools may lead some students to become passive but, as we alluded to above, it can also lead to even more problematic responses. As we said, it can produce an exaggerated performance of some of masculinity's most negative traits—reacting quickly and forcefully to challenges of any kind, a hypersensitivity to even insignificant affronts, and an extreme investment in the appearance of control and "cool" detachment. When these masculinized reactions predominate, they can change the atmosphere in alternative high schools in ways that are also detrimental to the Latinas with whom the young men interact. The masculinized atmosphere of aggressive display and physicality can intimidate girl students and interfere with their learning process. The following exchange derived from field notes was not uncommon at GCHS, where forms of verbal or physical aggression occurred on a daily basis.

> June [the classroom teacher who is white] walks over to the tall boy [Latino] at the computer and he notices her coming,
> "Oh my gosh. Please come over and hassle me," he says sarcastically.
> "You're supposed to be reading," begins June.
> "I am!" he insists loudly, "Are you trying to get rid of me, June?"
> June tells him to go outside. He exclaims in frustration, "Jesus H. Christ!" and June heads out the classroom door ahead of him . . . . he goes to pick up his backpack at the table and another boy in the class [who is white] yells, "Fuck the system!" and raises both his middle fingers as the tall boy begins picking up his notebook to put in his backpack. He yells loudly, "Am I getting a referral for making my fucking point!?" and storms out of the classroom.

The most common ways these disruptions occurred in daily interactions at GCHS usually involved profanity and defiance toward teachers, and at times even the volunteers. The eruptions were mostly the result of the acting out by boys of all races and ethnicities. In comparison, girls, the majority of whom were Latinas, expressed their defiance by passively resisting directions but almost always ending up complying. Instead of public disobedience, many Latina students would complain to each other about teachers but rarely if ever openly defied them.

The disruption and defiance observed at schools like GCHS sometimes escalate into something more severe. According to a national youth study, students in alternative high schools are at a greater risk of injury through violence than students in mainstream schools. The results indicate that, whereas 62.3% of students in alternative high schools had engaged in at least one physical fight in the last 12 months, only 36.6% had done so in mainstream high schools (Grunbaum, Lowry, & Kann, 2001). Unfortunately, the results were not broken down by race, ethnicity, and gender.

At GCHS, staff attempted to modify aggressive and defiant displays by disciplining students in various ways, including subjecting them to verbal warnings and sending students to the principal's office. They also issued "contracts" for such actions as making rude comments, using profanity, and other inappropriate behaviors. Contracts are the school's highest form of disciplinary action and require a parental conference with the student and teacher. During contract meetings, participants identify the problem and discuss possible ways to improve the student's behavior. Students are given three formal warnings and a hearing before potential expulsion. In addition, "referrals" were given out for the use of cell phones on the school premises.

The school's "no tolerance policy" for cell phone infractions was difficult to enforce, despite daily cell phone confiscations.

Although we found a gender difference in open displays of defiance among young women and men attending GCHS, young Latinas were none-theless affected by these displays. In effect, women are perceived by the larger society as less dangerous than men: They earn less, they are victimized more, and they do most of the emotional and social reproductive labor nec-essary for society to survive (women head most single households with chil-dren present). The open defiance exhibited mostly by boys at GCHS—not only because of gender socialization but also because of their numerical superiority—resulted in Latina students becoming part of the background and not receiving as much attention. However well intentioned teachers were at GCHS, the eruptions caused by the young men distracted them from providing full support to young women in their classes (from field notes):

> Once Juana [a Latina student] finishes her assignment, she tries to get June's [the classroom teacher] attention. It takes Juana raising her hand and saying June's name a few times to get her attention. June appears distracted, and more focused and concerned about helping the boys. This becomes apparent when June tells Juana just to have me [the eth-nographer] check her work. Juana then turns to me but I think she would have preferred to have had June's final say on her assignment.

The treatment Juana received from the teacher is in spite of the fact that girls at GCHS as a group took the assigned schoolwork more seriously than the boys and were more likely to complete their assignments. Many times their dedication and discipline was eclipsed by the boys' boisterous and aggres-sive behavior.

GENDERED MICROAGGRESSIONS

In addition to witnessing aggressive behavioral displays—sometimes ones severe enough to disrupt the classroom and impair their learning—Latina students suffered significant psychological stress and trauma as a result of the gendered "microaggressions" they experienced. "Microaggressions" are subtle but hurtful forms of day-to-day social interactions in which persons feel demeaned and degraded in ways that create psychological discomfort. According to Pierce (1995), microaggressions are defined as:

> subtle, innocuous, preconscious, or unconscious degradations, and put-downs, often kinetic but capable of being verbal and/or kinetic. In and of itself a micro-aggression may seem harmless, but the cumulative burden of a lifetime of microaggressions can theoretically contribute to dimin-ished mortality, augmented morbidity, and flattened confidence. (p. 281)

They are often brief—even momentary—commonplace verbal, behavioral, and environmental "slights," typically directed at marginalized persons by dominant group members. Microaggressions occur in everyday interactions and happen in many mundane contexts. They may be expressed in comments (such as a male calling another male a "girl" or "sissy"), in subtle snubs or exclusions (such as being ignored in class, or being avoided by the staff), or through dismissive looks, gestures, or tones. They are sometimes intentional and sometimes not, but nonetheless produce negative psychological reactions in those persons who are their targets or recipients. Although microaggressions may seem superficially harmless, their effects can accumulate over time; daily and extended exposure can produce serious mental health consequences (such as depression).

Not surprisingly, microaggessions are "probably the most grievous of offensive mechanisms spewed at victims of racism and sexism" (Pierce, 1995, p. 281). Our ethnographic research suggests that they are commonly experienced by Latina alternative high school students. Among other things, the gender- and ethnicity-specific norms of hyper-monitoring in these settings means that they regularly feel "under watch." They become hyper-vigilant and scared to exercise their own agency. Some retreat into reactance and become increasingly reluctant to follow rules and school structure. Heightened surveillance, negative judgments, the differential enforcement of rules, and disproportionately harsh sanctions all constitute microaggressions that students of color more commonly experience. Microaggressions administered by authority figures in highly structured school environments where Latino students already feel marginalized can parallel the process of prisonization, forcing them to adopt strategies of psychological survival that, in turn, prepare them for (and lead them to expect) various forms of incarcerative social and institutional control. The same carceral mentality and adaptations that are required to survive in such highly monitored environments also resemble some of the survival strategies that are required in vulnerable, poor communities of color.

The effects of microaggressions are cumulative but difficult to measure. We found that young Latinas, especially, were not encouraged to notice, react to, or talk about such microaggressions. Thus, they had few if any opportunities to reflect on or discuss such experiences, let alone acknowledge the damage they might incur. There was no emotional discourse with which to label these experiences, and no intellectual or therapeutic framework to assess and work through their consequences. Unlike women in higher education who have access to a language and a set of concepts through which to understand and process the microaggressions to which they are subjected—sexual harassment, date rape, and sexism—the young Latinas at CGHS did not. Whatever their injuries, they were largely suffered in silence and remained invisible.

Moreover, they sometimes occurred in such a way that there was little or nothing the Latina students could do to protect themselves. In some cases, the microaggressions were directed at them not only by their male peers but even by otherwise committed school staff. A poignant example occurred in class when two very dedicated teachers, June and Joe, decided to combine their classes into a "Socratic Seminar" designed to teach media literacy (field notes):

> In preparation for the seminar the classroom seats were rearranged into a rectangle so students could face each other and exchange ideas. As is usual in many classrooms, the students self-segregated by gender, with most of the young men sitting together and the young women following the same pattern (only one young white woman was present and she sat with the Latinas). The teachers followed suit with June sitting with the Latinas and Joe with the young men. The logic for the teachers' sitting arrangements was that June would join the Latinas to facilitate their participation in the discussion because they generally did not speak up in class. Joe had prepared a brief PowerPoint titled "Hip Hop: Beyond Beats and Rhymes. Socratic Seminar." He then encouraged students to pick a topic for discussion from the eight he had suggested. Immediately all the young men simultaneously clamored for different topics. The exchange devolved quickly with some of the boys shouting as a potential topic "Bitches and Hoes." Joe tried to calm the young men down by asking them if "the way music videos and the media are portraying women and calling them names is good for women." One of the young men mentioned a music video by the rapper 50 Cent and a woman being "credit carded," which entails a black man in a video sliding a credit card down a black woman's buttocks while she is wearing a thong bikini (the video is actually by hip hop rapper Nelly and the song is "Tip Drill") (slacktimeTV, 2014). The young men were obviously familiar with the video.

The video itself is so degrading to women that it is difficult to watch. It depicts as many as thirty black women in thong bikinis in a mansion having sexual exchanges with each other in a Jacuzzi and poolside while black rappers throughout the video throw bills at them. Yet, in the discussion that ensued, young men of all ethnicities and races claimed that women were not being exploited as long as they agreed to participate and were getting paid. With one exception, the Latina students remained silent and did not participate in the discussion. In fact, one Latina student and one white woman student agreed with the young men that it was the women's choice to be "credit carded." As recorded in the field notes:

> One boy says that she [the Black woman being "credit carded"] wanted to do it so why not. Joe asks them if they think this is proper treatment for a woman. Another boy in class says, "Yeah, otherwise she

wouldn't be doing it." One boy jokingly asks another if he'd want to be credit carded, he deflects the question and says, "Why would I want someone to do that?" At this point Joe realizes the boys are monopolizing the conversation and asks the boys to quiet down and let the girls speak. "Yeah, girls, speak. Don't be shy," says a blondish brown haired boy with short hair and a dark gray shirt. "C'mon girls, what do you think?" says the black male in a white shirt and black baseball cap. The girls don't say anything, and look at each other awkwardly. The boys don't wait patiently for long and once again start talking. The only white female in the group answers, "She's getting paid." The boys, liking this answer, start agreeing. A Latina girl whose dark hair is held up in a bun with her hands tucked inside her black pullover sweater finally says, "Well, it's her body and she's getting paid for it," supporting the white girl's answer. The Black boy makes a comment about how in Greek mythology Zeus created women as a punishment to men. June decides to intervene in the conversation, questioning the types of jobs they're getting paid to do. The Black boy tells June that she has a job and "Why you complaining," since he thinks the girls in the video want to be doing what they're doing and are even getting paid for it.

The discussion takes another turn

when the boys begin talking about women's behavior and how sometimes they want boys to "grab some cake." The Black youth, who has been very vocal about what he thinks women want, comments that boys want to "grab cake" and if the girl dresses in certain ways it's obvious that it's okay for them to "grab her cake." A Latino boy dressed in a flannel black and grey long sleeved shirt, with shaggy black hair mentions, "Yeah, what boy doesn't want to grab cake," and demonstrates by slapping one hand with the other.

The degrading "grab cake" imagery is likely a reference to a hip hop video by popular singer Rihanna, where she points to her genital region as offering "her cake" (Pop Archive, 2012). The video was entitled "Birthday Cake" and, although it shows Rihanna as very much in charge throughout, it also includes hyper-sexualized visuals depicting her and her on and off boyfriend, Chris Brown who, in fact, had been incarcerated for having physically assaulted her. In this context, the male student's assertion that women freely choose hypersexualization and readily grant permission to "grab their cake" is more easily understood. But there was no room for the girls to disagree. Except for the two girls who supported the boys in the discussion, the Latinas remained silent. Even when Joe encouraged them to speak, they found it difficult to find their footing in the highly charged, aggressive discussion that was dominated by the young men.

Joe tried to further the young men's views by asking them how would "they really know" that young women want to be touched in that way.

> The Black youth and a white youth with shaggy blond hair, in a black shirt, sporting a few silver chains both agree that it's based on what the girl is wearing. The other boys nod in agreement. They continue saying that some girls wear it because they want that kind of attention and if she didn't she wouldn't giggle and smile, and if she didn't like it, she would just get mad, but that it was definitely down to what she was wearing. The white female again comments that she agrees it would be the girl's "own fault." "Be honest, now ladies," says the Black youth [male] and expectantly looks at the girls' side of the room. The girls again are timid and don't really answer, the Latina girl in the black sweater speaks up again and says that "Yeah, but that's not the only thing they care about."

Joe tries to rescue the discussion by offering an alternative view of what girls are feeling:

> Joe brings up the point that women are not first seen for their intelligence and are instead only seen as hypersexualized. He asks the group why they think that is? The entire time Joe is speaking the boys are still arguing about how the girls won't answer their question. The white male in the bright blue cap says, "It's not the right group" because the girls aren't talking or commenting. Joe raises his voice to be heard above them and says that the boys are doing plenty of saying but not enough listening. He then turns their comments on them by asking, "If personality is what matters, why do girls feel the need to dress a certain way?" The Latina girl wearing a knitted dark magenta sweater who had sat on the boys' side tries to speak over the boys' comments. At this point the boys and the few girls on the other side of the room that are commenting are saying that it's because the girls want to and they want that kind of attention. Joe notices a girl trying to speak and quiets them. The girl says girls dress like that because that's what guys want. Joe points out that "She's saying that girls dress that way because guys want them to but you guys are saying that's not what guys want. How many of you guys have told a girl you don't have to dress like that? [to get my attention]. Girls has a guy ever told you that?" They're all momentarily quiet. . . . "I don't know, I just smoke weed," says the Latino youth in the flannel shirt, and then adds, "It's all on the girl." He turns and spits into the trashcan behind him.

Again Joe tries to rescue the discussion by stating: "I notice you have been placing all the blame on the women and this has a lot to do with the fact that men are the ones with the power." He is unsuccessful as one of the

white male students insists, "No, it's not" and that "it's a two way street."
Joe continues to try to convince them by stating, "It's not, and it goes back
to men having the control," but he is unsuccessful as the young man is still
not convinced, "I don't think men are too much in control." This entire time
the girls are silent in the overall discussion and so is the other teacher, June.
The bell rings and Joe says as a final remark "that he is troubled by their
seminar since it seems media messages are working since men are able to
place all the blame on women."

Thus, even this otherwise well-intentioned attempt to raise consciousness by two of the dedicated teachers at the school devolved into something
else. The microaggressions were not subtle, especially from the perspective
of 16 and 17-year-old girls. The images in the video itself verged on sexual
violence (one reinforced by the subtext that Rihanna herself had been physically assaulted by her boyfriend with whom she nonetheless appeared in
a hypersexualized video). Ironically, both Chris Brown and Rihanna were
not much older than the students in the class when the assault took place.
In addition, although the class was designed to examine sexism and sexual
violence, it included borderline pornographic images of black women (no
similar portrayals of white women were included or discussed), and the discussion itself was conducted primarily by a white male teacher. None of the
women in the room, including June, actively participated in the discussion
and, of the three women who spoke at all, two fully supported the young
men's point of view.

There is another dimension to these gendered microaggressions. Many of
the Latina students at GCHS come from poor, immigrant, and farm worker
families. GCHS is located in a fairly rural area of Northern California. As
such, the urban, youth black culture represented in the videos discussed may
not be as familiar to the Latina students as it might be to urban youth.
The two main videos discussed actually come with a warning label because
of the explicit lyrics and images (the lyrics so explicit that it is difficult to
justify printing them in this chapter). The discussion described above took
place in an English dominant classroom. Although the Latina students in this
class were fluent in English, many of their parents were not. The dominant
language in many of these homes is Spanish. It is difficult to imagine how
the Latina students could discuss the videos with their parents, unfamiliar
both with English and urban youth culture, or how they might translate the
notion of "credit carding" a woman or ask them whether they thought a
woman was inviting men to touch her "cake" by what she wore. This kind of
barrier between classroom experiences and the possibility of discussing especially troubling issues with their parents further alienates and marginalizes
Latina students, who have few other outlets through which to make sense of
the extreme objectification and sexual violence sanctioned in the materials
to which they were exposed. In exchanges like the one we described above,
they are often unable to fully articulate why their interactions with the young
men made them uncomfortable and unsettled. Such isolation is likely to add

to potential confusion, fear, and destabilization of Latina's views of their sexuality, control over their bodies, and their value as human beings.

We quoted and analyzed this exchange at length because we believe it encapsulates many aspects of the kind of gendered microaggressions to which Latinas are subjected. Also, not uncommonly, even dedicated teachers at this school seemed ill equipped to address the silencing of the Latina students' voices or remedy the structural masculinization of the classroom. These dynamics of male microaggressions in an explicitly masculinized classroom are especially harmful in alternative high schools where young Latinas are already marginalized by language, culture, class, sexuality, and gender. In predominantly male environments, like the ones that exist in many alternative schools, it becomes essential for young Latinas to have a "space of their own" to discuss the microaggressive interactions that expose them to psychological (and, potentially, even physical) violence.

In addition, it is important to note the ways in which these dynamics serve as precursors to those that are taken to more extreme levels in juvenile and adult correctional institutions, thus constituting another form of early prisonization. Young men of color, already marginalized enough by the system of public education to be placed in alternative schools, no doubt sense the troubled trajectory that the larger society has doomed them to travel. Many sense that their own autonomy, agency, and efficacy are in jeopardy, and the desire to assert a hegemonic masculinity in which they seek to enact exaggerated versions of manhood represents one form of compensation. It is a strategy that is too often taken to much more extreme levels in juvenile halls and adult prisons and jails, where young men are emasculated and infantilized by their conditions of confinement and frequently take refuge in a profoundly sexist culture. In part for these reasons, "hypermasculinity" and the corresponding maladies of misogyny and homophobia are pervasive in such places (e.g., Haney, 2011). But early exposure to highly masculinized institutional settings, such as alternative schools, provides boys and girls with a potentially destructive template for gender dynamics that many will encounter in a more pernicious form later in life.

CONCLUSION

Unfortunately, these dynamics are mostly invisible and seldom examined. It is rare that intersectional analyses are applied to alternative schools or other masculinized institutions like juvenile hall and jails. The topics are understudied in academia and often escape public and political commentary as well. For example, by contrast, much recent focus has centered on the consequences of criminalization on boys and young men of color. President Obama has rightly championed this cause by launching the "My Brother's Keeper Initiative" (MBK), whose purpose is to "take a collaborative and multidisciplinary approach to building ladders of opportunity for boys and young men of Color" ("FACT SHEET: Opportunity for all: President Obama Launches My Brother's Keeper Initiative to Build Ladders of Opportunity For Boys and Young Men of Color," 2014, para. 11). MBK creates access to resources from a young age for this population by increasing parental involvement, ameliorating the disciplinary process in education, and collaborating with the criminal justice system to better intervene and create positive futures. The mission is to identify agencies and programs in the community, businesses, and elected officials and utilize these resources to improve the outcomes for young men of color. The hope is to advance the achievement of young men of color who are most at risk and the least likely to attend college and build a career.

However, when compared to young white women, young women of color are also disproportionately affected by criminalization. As Kimberle Crenshaw (2014) and a group of academics wrote in reaction to President Obama's "My Brother Keeper's Initiative:"

> While we applaud the efforts on the part of the White House, private philanthropy, social justice organizations and others to move beyond colorblind approaches to race-specific problems, we are profoundly troubled about the exclusion of women and girls of color from this critical undertaking. The need to acknowledge the crisis facing boys should not come at the expense of addressing the stunted opportunities for girls who live in the same households, suffer in the same schools, and struggle to overcome a common history of limited opportunities caused by various forms of discrimination. (para. 2)

Troubled by the exclusion of girls, Crenshaw and her colleagues pled the case for President Obama to acknowledge and address their plight as well. She highlighted key similarities in education and vulnerabilities in the justice system that consistently overlap with the barriers their male counterparts face, along with the economic barriers specific to women. Crenshaw ended her appeal by critiquing the lack of an intersectional lens used to address these challenges. She urged President Obama to focus on the "shared fate" of people of color and to instead improve their communities as a whole. Furthermore, Crenshaw pointed to the lack of evidence in justifying the decision not also to focus on young women of color:

> Our daughters are ignored and under-researched. Although the exclusion of girls has been justified as data-driven, the fact is that little data is gathered on them. This situation creates a vicious cycle in which the assumption that girls are not in crisis leads to research and policy interventions that overlook them. (para. 10)

The lack of focus on young women of color can be translated to the experiences of young Latinas in alternative education. In these spaces they are also often overlooked and are rarely central in the analysis (Malagon & Alvarez, 2010) despite increasingly entering the same disenfranchised institutions that men of color populate. The critical lens must be broadened to include the lived realities of young Latinas in masculinized institutions.

NOTE

1 In compliance with the agreement between the ethnographer and the school, the identities of the school, teachers, and the students has been kept confidential and pseudonyms have been used in substitution of their real names.

REFERENCES

Alternative Education (About). (2008). Retrieved June 24, 2014, from http://www.doe.mass.edu/alted/about.html?section=definition
Accrediting Commission for Schools, Western Association of Schools and Colleges. (2009). *The Grove Continuation School WASC Report*. Burlingame, CA: Accrediting Commission for Schools.
Bandura, A. (1995). *Self-efficacy in changing societies*. Cambridge, MA: Cambridge University Press.
California Department of Education. (2014). *DataQuest*. Retrieved from http://dq.cde.ca.gov/dataquest/
California Department of Education. (2013). *Fingertip Facts on Education in California, CalEdFacts*. Retrieved from http://www.cde.ca.gov/ds/sd/cb/ceffingertipfacts.asp
Carver, P. R., Lewis, L., & Tice, P. (2010). *Alternative schools and programs for public school students at risk of educational failure: 2007–08. First Look* (NCES 2010-026). National Center for Education Statistics.
Collins, P. H. (2002). *Black feminist thought*. New York: Routledge.
Corbett, C., Hill, C., & St. Rose, A. (2008). *Where the girls are: The facts about gender equity in education*. Washington, DC: American Association of University Women Educational Foundation..
Collins, P. H. (2002). *Black feminist thought*. New York: Routledge.
County QuickFacts from the US Census Bureau. (2014, June 11). Retrieved from http://quickfacts.census.gov/.html
Crenshaw, K. (2014). Letter from women of color urging inclusion of women and girls in MBK. [Petition]. African American Policy Forum: New York, NY.
http://www.aapf.org/recent/2014/06/woc-letter-mbk
Emerson, R. M., Fretz, R. I., & Shaw, L. L. (2011). *Writing ethnographic fieldnotes*. Chicago: University of Chicago Press.
Fact Sheet: Opportunity for all: President Obama Launches My Brother's Keeper Initiative to Build Ladders of Opportunity for Boys and Young Men of Color. (2014, February 27). The White House. Retrieved from http://www.whitehouse.gov/the-press-office/2014/02/27/fact-sheet-opportunity-all-president-obama-launches-my-brother-s-keeper-
Fetterman, D. M. (2010). *Ethnography: Step-by-step*. Los Angeles: SAGE.
Fine, M., & Weis, L. (1998). *The unknown city*. Boston: Beacon Press.
Gable, R. A., Bullock, L. M., & Evans, W. H. (2006). Changing perspectives on alternative schooling for children and adolescents with challenging behavior. *Preventing School Failure: Alternative Education for Children and Youth, 51*(1), 5–9.

Grunbaum, J. A., Lowry, R., & Kann, L. (2001). Prevalence of health-related behaviors among alternative high school students as compared with students attending regular high schools. *Journal of Adolescent Health, 29*(5), 337–343.

Haney, C. (2003). The psychological impact of incarceration: Implications for post-prison adjustment. In J. Travis & M. Waul (Eds.), *Prisoners once removed. The impact of incarceration and reentry on children, families, and communities* (pp. 33–66). Washington, DC: The Urban Institute.

Haney, C. (2011). The perversions of prison: On the origins of hypermasculinity and sexual violence in confinement. *American Criminal Law Review, 48*, 121–141.

Haney, C., and Zimbardo, P. (1973). Social roles, role-playing, and education: On the high school as prison. *The Behavioral and Social Science Teacher, 1*, 24–45.

Hirschfield, P. (2008). Preparing for prison? The criminalization of school discipline in the USA. *Theoretical Criminology, 12*, 79–101.

Hurtado, A. (1996). *The color of privilege: Three blasphemies on race and feminism.* Ann Arbor: University of Michigan Press.

Hurtado, A. (2003). *Voicing Chicana feminisms: Young Chicanas speak out on sexuality and feminism.* New York: New York University Press.

Hurtado, A. (2010). Multiple lenses: Multicultural feminist theory. In H. Landrine & N. F. Russo (Eds.), *Handbook of diversity in feminist psychology* (pp. 29–54). New York: Springer.

Hurtado, A., & Cervantez, K. (2009). A view from within and from without. In F. A. Villarruel, G. Carlo, J. Grau, M. Azmitia, N. Cabrera & T. J. Chahin, (Eds.), *Handbook of US Latino Psychology: Developmental and Community-Based Perspectives* (pp. 171–190). Thousand Oakes, CA: Sage Publications.

Hurtado, A., Haney, C. W., & Hurtado, J. (2012). Where the boys are: Macro and micro considerations for the study of young latino men's educational achievement. In P. Noguera, A. Hurtado, & E. Fergus. *Understanding the disenfranchisement of Latino men and boys: Invisible no more* (pp. 102–121). New York: Routledge.

Hurtado, A., & Sinha, M. (in press). *Beyond Machismo: Intersectional understandings of Latinos' feminist masculinities.* Austin, TX: University of Texas Press.

Lange, C. M., & Sletten, S. J. (2002). *Alternative education: A brief history and research synthesis.* Retrieved from http://www.sde.idaho.gov/site/alternative_chools/docs/alt/alternative_ed_history%202002.pdf

Lehr, C. A., Tan, C. S., & Ysseldyke, J. (2009). Alternative Schools: A Synthesis of State-Level Policy and Research. *Remedial and Special Education, 30*(1), 19–32.

Lofland, J., & Lofland, L. H. (1995). *Analyzing social settings: A guide to qualitative observation and analysis.* Belmont, CA: Wadsworth.

Malagon, M. C. (2010). All the losers go there: Challenging the deficit educational discourse of Chicano racialized masculinity in a continuation high school. *Educational Foundations, 24*(1), 18–18.

Malagon, M. C., & Alvarez, C. R. (2010). Scholarship girls aren't the only Chicanas who go to college: Former Chicana continuation high school students disrupting the educational achievement binary. *Harvard Educational Review, 80*(2), 149–173.

Parsons, R. (2013). Keepin' It Movin': Portraits from a New York City transfer school. *Schools: Studies in Education, 10*(1), 59–71.

Pierce, C. M. (1995). Stress analogs of racism and sexism: Terrorism, torture, and disaster. In C. V. Willie, P. P. Rieker, B. M. Kramer, & B. S. Brown (Eds.), *Mental health, racism, and sexism* (pp. 277–293). Pittsburgh: University of Pittsburgh Press.

Pop Archive. (2012, June 28). *Rihanna ft. Chris Brown-Birthday Cake remix Music Video* [Video file]. Retrieved from http://youtu.be/2_03U8zl5IE

Raywid, M. A. (1981). The first decade of public school alternatives. *Phi Delta Kappan, 62*, 551–554.

Sáenz, V. B., & Ponjuan, L. (2009). The vanishing Latino male in higher education. *Journal of Higher Education, 8*, 54–89. doi:10.1177/1538192708326995

Seligman, M. E. P. (1975). Helplessness: On depression, development, and death. San Francisco, CA: W. H. Freeman.

slacktimeTV. (2014). *Music video: Nelly-tip drill uncut* [Video file]. Retrieved from http://slack-time.com/music-video-2717-nelly-tip-drill

Valenzuela, A. (1999). "Checkin'up on My Guy": Chicanas, Social Capital, and the Culture of Romance. *Frontiers: A Journal of Women Studies, 20*, 60–79.

7 Disability and Silences That Do Not Tell

Linda Ware and Danielle Cowley

Cultural messages about sex and disability reinforce the binary construct of people with disabilities as either asexual innocents who cannot have sex, or at the other extreme, as hypersexualized beings who, unless their sexuality is contained and discouraged, will, as adults, pose a menace to society. In the example of intellectual disability, Desjardins (2012) cites from Block (2000) the history of two "rival" images that have been used to legitimize the "containment of the sexuality of these people: the seraphic idiot and the Mephistophelic idiot" (p. 67). Desjardins, drawing on the work of disability historians and social scientists, suggests it was during industrialization that the dominant traits of asexuality and depraved sexuality gained cultural currency in the example of intellectually disabled individuals.

Categorization schemes derived by medicine and social work strived to delineate the degree of deviancy from an imagined norm, in an effort to protect the angelic idiot from the dangers of sexuality, while other factions wanted to protect society from the lasciviousness and the "vices of demonic idiot" (Desjardins, 2012, p. 70). He noted, drawing from the disability historian Henri Stiker (1996), three socially imposed measures to resolve society's concerns: institutionalization, eugenic sterilization, and later, special education. Snyder and Mitchell (2006) attribute this period of "Western modes of intolerance toward biologically based differences" (p. 113) to trends of scientific management that established the context for eugenics. Further, they underscore that the outcome of the obsession with classification systems during this era gave rise to "nearly all the disciplinary arenas that are today responsible for the management and oversight of people with disabilities, including medicine, therapy, charity, special education, social work, psychology, psychiatry, institutional administration and policy" (Snyder & Mitchell, 2006, p. 113). Arguably, much of this was based on human capital theory and market productivity.

It was during this period when obsessive human classification schemes produced scientific terminology such as "idiots," "morons," or "feeble-mindedness." This launched the continued cataloging of individuals as "biological outcasts" (Snyder & Mitchell, 2006). They note of this period that one "era's 'scientific' designations become another era's derogatory epithets" (Snyder & Mitchell, 2006, pp. 18–19). What we are left with as a society today is the inability to view human variation free of subjective judgment and cultural meaning systems rooted in the past. Regardless of the disability, what follows is a generalized morphing of the body that is perceived as disabled into a sexual binary that is viewed as abnormal at either extreme and outside the sphere where access to sexuality and reproduction is socially permitted.

In this chapter, we explore the value of launching a conversation on sex and disability with educators, staff, and school administrators informed by a disability studies framework. We include contributions from the arts, disability theorists, and the voices of young women. Although the silences we consider are plural, authored by multiple individuals in various locations, and not exclusively by educators, it is our contention that K-12 educational settings serve as the most critical cultural space in which to challenge the silence on disability sexuality.

TO HUNGER

> Sex and disability are two words that you don't often hear together and if you do, it's like . . . "those people have sex?"
>
> Maria Palacios, *Sins Invalid* (Berne, 2013)

Maria Palacios, a poet and dancer with the San Francisco-based *Sins Invalid* performance troupe, delves into the "abnormality" of disability sexuality in her art, including her spoken word piece entitled "Hunger" featured in the documentary, *Sins Invalid* (Berne, 2013). Palacios is a physically vibrant performer who wheels across the stage, rousing the audience to recognize the injustice of a young woman's future foreclosed by social norms. "Hunger" is raw and revealing on many levels, as it informs contemporary cultural perceptions about disability and sexual identity authored by those who live the experience. Reconstructed from memories excavated from her youth, Palacios, who is physically disabled, occupies the same cultural frame described by Desjardins, as her claims to sexuality and desire are taboo. Palacios describes her survival in a family that was ill-prepared to guide her through desire and sexual exploration on the way to defining her womanhood. She was burdened by the belief she would never have sex, marry if she wanted to, and never have children. Simply put, she was issued an edict to never grow up. Today Palacious draws from those memories to fuel her passion and her presentation of a woman who is confident and candid about her sexuality.

SURVIVE, BUT NEVER GROW UP

The Chicago-based visual artist and disability activist Riva Lehrer reflects on her adolescence and the influence of the frame her family placed on her in "Golem Girl Gets Lucky" (2012):

> I was a frozen child in my mother's house. She was frantic to protect me from what might happen when and if I did grow up. After she tried so hard to help me survive, the future slowed down and became a place where I was not allowed to ripen. My puberty threatened to elide straight into Sleeping Beauty's cryogenic coma. She tried to keep me in her maternal stronghold so that I could remain unthreatened by the desires of men. (Lehrer, 2012, p. 236)

Lehrer recalled that as a child, her mother sewed clothing identical to her own, and from the remnants, doll costumes to match. For years Lehrer beamed with pride for "those outfits, and looking just like Mommy" (p. 236). However, in adolescence the cruel consequences of infantilizing Lehrer, as if she was a doll on display, seemed to reverse direction to a sort of 'hiding' by the family in response to the onset of her physical development as a young woman:

> [I]t was clear that everyone—Dad, Grandma, Grandpa, Aunt Ruth, Aunt Sarah, Uncle Barry, Uncles Lester, all my cousins, doctors, nurses, teachers, housekeepers, neighbors, milkmen and the Rabbi—all agreed that my safest place was in hiding. (p. 236)

When Lehrer's mother discovered a locket with the yearbook picture of a boy, her 'crush' became a joke to family members who teased Lehrer into the belief that the potential for such a relationship was "something totally bizarre and inappropriate" (p. 239). That Lehrer's 'crush' might have been typical adolescent girl behavior was beyond the realm of possibility according to those who loved her. It was unimaginable that Lehrer would author a life of healthy sexual exploration and disability identity development explored through her art and in solidarity with numerous disability communities worldwide. But she did.

"TOO MUCH TO EXPECT"

Don't Call Me Inspirational, A Disabled Feminist Talks Back, by Harilyn Rousso (2013), a noted New York City-based disability activist, feminist, psychotherapist, writer, and painter, takes up sex and disability dilemmas similar to those posed by Palacios and Lehrer. Rousso recalls the impact of 1970s activism when the intersection of various civil rights movements proved personally relevant for dismantling identity claims relative to gender, sexuality, and disability rights. Upon reflection it was a time that prompted the recognition for Rousso that "I didn't have to pretend I was nondisabled anymore. And for the first time, I was not the only one in the group with a disability" (p. 6). She advanced awareness of the need to include adolescents and women with disabilities in larger conversations about living in a social milieu that too often excluded them.

Despite the socially conscious context of the 1970s in which Rousso began to explore her identity as a woman with disabilities, the pretense, hiding, non-disclosure, and silence that marked her adolescent years remained very much a part of her sense of self throughout her life. Today, she lives a vibrant life shaped by family, friends, and professional recognition, yet what she discovered in the memoir writing process roused revelations long silenced. In the short story "Adolescent Conversation," Russo wondered, "Why didn't I talk about my disability with my best friends during adolescence?" "What would I have said?" (2013, p. 41). In an imagined exchange on disability, identity, and sexuality with Elaine, her best friend, she described herself as "lucky" because her Cerebral Palsy was "really a mild case. . . . You know I can do everything." Elaine, her non-disabled friend, asked, "Can you have sex?" Harilyn, unsure, replied, "I think I can . . . [but] I would be too embarrassed to ask. . . . Anyhow, who would want to 'have sex' with me?" (p. 41). Having spent years as an activist, Rousso hoped her memoir on this exchange might become a resource to inform the mentorship of adolescent girls:

> If only I could spare them that self-hatred, secrecy, silence—help them see that there is nothing wrong with who they are, as they are, disability and all, that they can have a satisfying life with their disability, and not despite it. Too much to expect from young girls who feel they must hide so much of themselves to get through their lives. (p. 204)

MOVING BEYOND PITY OR FEAR—BUILDING A CURRICULUM

Inviting educators into a conversation on disability sexuality informed by the work of Palacious, Lehrer, and Rousso would be challenging on many levels. One obvious obstacle would be to stress that the physical disabilities experienced by the individuals we consider here are not assumed to map onto the experiences of individuals with intellectual disabilities. In addition, it would be our hope that an exploration with educators, community members, and parents/caregivers would begin with honest recognition of participant biases and assumptions. If the goal is truly to explore curriculum that exceeds the parameters of pity or fear, the struggle to recognize complexity must be a given. An additional challenge is informed by the research of Griffiths and Lunsky (2000), who indicate that attitudes today may be even more negative toward sexual relationships and marriages of people with intellectual disabilities than compared to 20 years ago.

In an effort to explain this seeming regressive turn, we draw on Desjardins' (2012) notion of society's "veiled margins" in the instance of intellectual disabilities. In effect, this amounts to the unintended consequences of "normalization" efforts that provide intellectually disabled youth living options in "parallel communities" (p. 83). In his research, youth were observed for a period of 24 months in settings designed to "initiate them to normal life and to integrate them within global society" beneath the banner of rehabilitative, transition experiences (Desjardins, 2012, p. 83). Desjardins found instead what amounted to a parody of integration wherein the participants he observed essentially "mimicked, as best they could, the ways and customs of the majority of the population; and their transition from otherness to normality, within the confines of these veiled margins [that] will never end" (p. 84). He suggested that their "otherness" is hidden in plain sight, albeit veiled behind signifiers of normality. In much the same way that Lehrer recalled, "the future slowed down and became a place where I was not allowed to ripen" (p. 236), Dejardins' research indicated that the coerced sterilization of young women with intellectual disabilities—in the name of "good choices"—was orchestrated by family members.

The rhetorical history of normativity props up conventional constructs relative to sexual identities among people with disabilities whether the disability is physical or intellectual. That is, regardless of the disability category and whether the disability is visible or invisible, difference is marked on the body and that proves problematic relative to sexual identity and claims to sexual expression (Garland-Thomson, 1996; Gill, 2015; Linton 1998, 2003; Snyder & Mitchell, 2006). The editors of the recently published *Sex and Disability* (2012), Robert McRuer and Anna Mollow, note:

> When sex and disability are linked in contemporary American cultures, the conjunction is most often the occasion for marginalization or marveling: the sexuality of disabled people is typically depicted in terms of either tragic deficiency or freakish excess. Pity or fear, in other words, are the sensations most often associated with disabilities; more pleasurable sexual sensations are generally dissociated from disabled bodies and lives. (p. 1)

In order to fight the stigma of the sexually problematic status of people with disabilities, Wilkerson (2011) urges a commitment to recognize that "sexuality, as sexual identity, is one among a variety of axes of oppression" (p. 36). Among academics this might seem like a reasonable starting point to shift awareness, but among educators, this argument would likely prove to be highly controversial and politically combustible. Although many educators readily claim to support the development of empowered identity among students, sexual identity development remains overlooked and under-addressed. Ideally, educators would design curriculum locally and in the context of the students they teach. In the likely absence of understanding disability and sexuality outside the extreme poles of "pity and fear," many educators continue to suppress sexual agency and the freedom to author a fully empowered identity. Our goal is not to take educators to task. Rather, we hope by providing insights drawn from the experiences of visual artists and writers with disabilities, those who theorize disability and sexuality will launch a long overdue conversation in relation to schooling.

DISABILITY AND SEXUAL JUSTICE—"IT'S NOT A MATTER OF MORE RIGHTS"

As a young activist, the disability studies scholar Anne Finger (1992) was among the first wave of critics who challenged the silence on disability and sexual agency. She pointedly reminded us that the conversation on sexual agency would be as challenging for disabled people to enter as it might be for non-disabled people to imagine:

> Sexuality is often the source of our deepest oppression; it is also often the source of our deepest pain. It's easier for us to talk about—and for-mulate strategies for changing—discrimination in employment, educa-tion, and housing than to talk about our exclusion from sexuality and reproduction. (p. 9)

Similar to Rousso, Finger offers her perspective as an adult informed by memories of her early disability experience and disability rights activism in the 1970s. Armed with the nascent recognition of disability injustice as a civil rights issue, and poised in solidarity with those who made similar claims for race, gender, and sexual orientation equality, the emphasis on disability rights and the creation of legal mandates to ensure justice was a logical first step (Charlton, 2000; Colker 2005; Linton, 1998, 2006). More recently, Finger suggests disability sexuality requires a more nuanced and complex discourse informed by "more than rights" (McRuer & Mollow, 2012). She contends that in the present, sexual justice for disabled people is more likely to be influenced by the writing, painting, dance, and perfor-mance work of contemporary disability-inspired artists including Eli Clare, Terry Galloway, Riva Lehrer, and troupes such as *Sins Invalid* and *Axis Dance Company*.

Finger (2012) and Rousso (2013) suggest a cultural shift is needed that would encourage society to recognize the 'untold' desires that have figured into the lives of disabled people. Much of this critical work is recounted in contemporary memoirs, poetry, and performance. However, it is also cru-cial to politicize sex and disability in the broadest cultural space possible in pursuit of advancing disability theory. The section that follows builds on these issues framed in an educational context. In particular, what happens to the inclusive education model in education when disability and sexual agency become a part of the conversation?

INQUIRY VS. THE "LOCAL AND LIMITED"

As disability studies in education scholars and educators who prepare teachers to work in K-12 settings, it bears mention that our content and approach should not be confused with special education. We are among a growing number of teacher educators who have, over several decades, challenged the field of special education to become self-critical of discursive practices (Artiles, 2005; Ashby, 2012; Baglieri, Valle, Connor & Gallagher, 2011; Baker, 2002; Blatt, 1984; Ferri & Connor, 2013; Gallagher, Connor & Ferri, 2014; Hehir; 2005; Heshusius, 2004; Sktic, 1991; Ware, 2001, 2007, 2013). In brief, the distinction between disability studies in education and special education is that disability studies critiques special education's cure and remediation discourse on the basis that it undermines the status and self-regard of the individual with disability. We subscribe to a belief that does not locate deficiency. Simi Linton (2006), a well-respected disability activist frames the distinction succinctly noting that: "special education is not a solution to the 'problem' of disability, it *is* the problem, or at least one of the major impediments to the full integration of disabled people in society" (p. 161).

When we introduce disability studies as the intellectual home for courses, we underscore the need to adapt to models for teaching and understanding that fall outside of the typical special education training orientation (Ware, 2005, 2007, 2013). Inclusive education assumes this mindset, as noted by Oyler (2011) and others who advance the notion of teacher "inquiry" versus "knowledge and skills" as the starting point for inclusive educators working toward greater equity, more pluralism, and less oppression (p. 204). Inclusion in this context exceeds the "local and limited" understanding that erroneously equates the meaning of inclusion as "a place, not a set of services, and not a philosophy or approach" (Oyler, 2011, p. 205). Some thirty years following the roll out of inclusion in K-12 education, it remains a unique undertaking, more dependent on geography (i.e., a student's residence) than on the core values of the educational institution that would come to bear in efforts to define it. It should come as no surprise that educational inclusion has been met with resistance in public education by both general and special educators for multiple reasons (Ware, 2013). One roadblock is the failure to recognize disability as part of the spectrum of human difference (Biklen, 1988, 1992; Hehir, 2005; Ware, 2001, 2007). Disability studies in education begin with a grounding philosophy about disability as a cultural construct and as such, it is imperative to unpack the philosophical and ideological beliefs that inform practice and institutional organizations relative to disability (Gallagher et al., 2014; Oyler; 2011 Ware, 2004).

SEXUALITY IN A CULTURE OF SILENCE

When sexuality is discussed in K-12 educational settings, particularly in regard to young women with intellectual disabilities, the discourse is one of protection against violence or it is saturated with assumed heteronormativity (Abbott & Howarth, 2007; Anuos & Feldman, 2002; Parkes, 2006). Coupled with the potentially tumultuous years of adolescence, the sexuality of young women with intellectual or learning disabilities is shrouded in dangerous silence. Adolescents with disabilities—whether intellectual or physical—may experience negative self-image or experience difficulties developing intimate relationships, due in part to the stigma of their perceived differences (Gordon, Tschopp, & Feldman, 2004).

It was with this knowledge that one of us (Cowley, a white academic) interviewed four racially and economically diverse female students with disabilities. The interviews were conducted while the students worked on collage art projects. Data analysis involved coding and synthesizing into themes and looking for patterns and relationships (Bogdan & Biklen, 2006). A feminist analytical framework (Madison, 2005) was used to explore gender and sexuality. Two of the narrative case studies created are considered below. It bears noting that these qualitative interviews were not originally framed as an exploration of disability identity or disability sexuality. The overarching research set out to explore the transition needs of female adolescents as they prepared to exit high school. As the participants imagined the future, they were quick to draw bold lines that connected transition to a heteronormative script where dating and marriage figured more prominently than gainful employment—the assumed goal for many transition programs.

Britany: Fighting for Her Sexuality. As a 19-year-old high school student with an intellectual disability, Britany's identity straddles the borders of childhood and adulthood. She, among the four young women who participated in Cowley's (2013) research, expressed the greatest comfort with her sexuality and a budding identity linked to sexualized representation. Her collages were plastered with hegemonic images of traditional femininity: teenage girls in dresses, handbags, makeup, 'tween' heartthrobs, and sexualized female bodies.

Britany was drawn to such representations of traditional gender norms and sexualized images, seemingly in response to the borders that her mother created around her daughter's developing womanhood. She was among the most monitored of the participants by her mother's apparent desire to shelter her daughter in the transition from girlhood to womanhood. In much the same way that Palacios, Lehrer, and Rousso recounted earlier in this chapter, the stronghold her mother placed on Britany's exploration of sexuality was a frequent source of tension and resentment. She was not allowed to watch television shows that her mother considered "particularly intense" such as *Pretty Little Liars* (ABC Family). This show, popular among high school students, revolves around high school cliques, the disappearance and death of a friend, and threatening text messages sent back and forth between the characters. Britany responded to her mother's censorship by accessing the program in secret on the Internet. She also had her Facebook and Twitter privileges taken away at various times during the course of the research by her mother. Britany also took issue with the fact that her mother expressed disapproval of her desire to have sex. No discussion of sexuality as a natural feature of human development during adolescence was afforded to Britany at home or at school. And no mention was made of this on her Individualized Education Plan (IEP) despite her obvious interest in her development as a desirable young woman.

It is unclear who might provide the space in Britany's life or schooling to engage her in productive dialogue about issues of sexuality and her own choices relative to sexuality. Whereas Rousso expressed a sense of shame when recalling her own high school years and questions about sexuality and desire, for Britany, it was the adults who resisted engaging her on this topic. Through the collages and the interviews, Britany constructed a gendered identity that simultaneously pushed back against the label of intellectual disability and at her mother's overprotection. She created, resisted, and occupied simultaneous spheres of girl/womanhood that were facilitated by media and technology that she accessed.

It is very telling that Britany recognized the ways in which this monitoring positioned her outside the realm of a typical teenager. Her awareness of her mother's surveillance strategies signaled her meta-consciousness relative to her disability. Her developing self might have benefited greatly from a structured, school-based curriculum that placed her life in a context worthy of exploring (Cowley, Gebb, & Guthrie, 2015).

Much of the critical research regarding sexuality, sexual relationships, and parenting by individuals with intellectual disabilities occurs outside the US (Aunos & Feldman, 2002; Liecester & Cooke, 2002; Parkes, 2006). This body of research indicates that able-bodied teachers, professionals, and parents continue to have negative and conservative attitudes toward people with intellectual disabilities and sexuality. For example, Aunos and Feldman (2002) found that "75% of parents surveyed were against their children marrying and raising children," whereas "a majority of parents were against marriage even if their child would use contraception" (p. 289). On a more troubling note, in his research with Canadian families, Desjardins (2012) reported on the coercive strategies deployed by parents to secure consent for sterilization of their daughters with intellectual disabilities in the name of "good choices." This research is contrary to the fact that the majority of people with mild intellectual disabilities want to marry and raise a child (Aunos & Feldman, 2002). It does not take into consideration transgression from the heteronormative marriage plot between a man and a woman. Disabled adolescents are left with little or no information about the variety of ways they might hope to couple in a physical and or romantic relationship. As Palacious indicated in her poem, "Hunger"—"sex and love" were confused as she explored her womanhood, a confusion attributed to the absence of conversation and knowledge about womanhood traced back to her adolescent years.

Victoria: Policing sexuality. Adolescent girls with disabilities struggle when claiming girlhood or womanhood due, in part, to oppressive societal attitudes that position them outside the boundaries of sex and gender—as perpetually childlike. Contrary to this reality, Victoria, who was identified with intellectual disabilities, was able actively to assemble an identity that reclaimed girl/womanhood, and made space for advocacy at her school as a survivor of sexual violence. After an altercation with a boy who pulled her into a school bathroom and forcibly kissed her against her wishes, Victoria was initially policed at her school under the guise of insuring her safety. Each morning she was met at the bus by her paraprofessional, escorted between all classes by an adult, and ate lunch with her teachers. Victoria was afforded little input on this plan, which in fact, conflicted with her desire to claim a confident sexual identity. Research by Chenoweth (1996) has shown that discourses and practices of overprotection, segregation, and compliance lead to more violence rather than prevent it.

Victoria spoke a great deal about her boyfriend Geoff, and his daily phone calls. They attended different schools and much of what they chatted about was their school day. They made plans to visit each other at their respective homes with support coordinated by their parents. In the process of Cowley's interviews, Victoria related she and Geoff sometimes "wrestle" and "do our love stuff and just do our thing." When queried about the meaning of her expression, Victoria replied, "It's our love thing where we have to kiss and all that stuff. And do something on our bodies."

Victoria's relationship with Geoff was clearly an important part of how she imagines her future life. At the conclusion of one interview, Cowley asked—given that this research was designed to consider the transition from high school into adult life—if there was anything else she wanted to share that was important to planning for her future. Victoria hoped she would continue being a "wonderful student," a "hard worker," and that "playing games and travelling" would be a part of her future. She added that continuing a romantic relationship was also of importance. In fact, among future living options, she states she would live with her current boyfriend Geoff, who would, by then, be her husband. It was with conviction that Victoria offered a narrative of interdependent living supported by an intimate partner.

Given that Victoria's family was very supportive of her relationship with Geoff and they are close friends with his parents, the potential for this relationship to thrive seems likely. However, it bears mention that certain policies such as the sexual capacity assessment (NYSARCA, 2007) hold the potential to oppress the sexual expression of people with intellectual disabilities. This assessment utilizes medical and psychological indicators to determine the viability for an individual to claim sexual agency. The state in which Victoria resides defines the following: "Any sexual contact between persons receiving services and others, or among persons receiving services, is considered to be sexual abuse unless the involved person(s) is a consenting adult" (NYSARCA, 2007). Professional 'expertise' is used to determine whether or not an individual has the capacity to engage in sexual activity. If through this 'expert' assessment an individual is deemed without capacity to consent, she cannot engage in sexual contact. If she does, an investigation must ensue and local authorities must be notified. Persons with intellectual disabilities are put in a position to prove their capacity through assessment and must earn the right to a sexual relationship.

In addition, current research on caregivers' negative attitudes toward sexual expression among disabled people could likewise threaten the potential reality of Victoria living with and marrying her current boyfriend. That is to say, Victoria would fare better in the future provided her parents remain supportive of her claims to sexual agency, whereas Britany might be better served by demonstrating that she has the capacity to engage in sexual activity irrespective of her parents' directives. These two young women provide a glimpse into the complexity that must be taken up by educators willing to support the development of a school-based curriculum that would afford students like Britany and Victoria the freedom to transition to adult lives in fuller ways.

CONCLUSION

> I have become a woman over time. I certainly would have rejected such a title in the beginning. It could precipitate my death. Consign me to an itty-bitty life.
>
> Simi Linton, *My Body Politic (2006)*

Because schools serve as the most logical site to broaden understanding about disability in general, it can be argued that through our silence we reify the patriarchal impulse for overprotection and subsequent infantalization of youth with disabilities. Our silence will not protect young people from predatory threats, nor will it truly ensure their development as human beings, free to choose disability identity and sexual identity because they have been provided information, resources, and role models. In preparing to write this chapter, we were stymied by our frustration in considering how such a conversation might begin in schools, knowing that teachers are rarely afforded the time to engage in deep study together on topics such as this. Sexuality, in general, is a topic that is silenced in schools except in relation to HIV/AIDS and disease. Surely, we can do better than that.

Schools are populated by youth with disabilities who are taking on a stronger presence in the school day, on their own terms, in much the same way that disabled people included here are claiming their right to be in the world—also on their own terms. YouTube videos present an endless feed of youth performances that are perfectly suited for use with young people in schools. The videos often figure disability, informed as we have discussed it here, through a counter-narrative informed by a cultural lens. Yet, the extant curriculum serves up stereotypical constructs of "monstrosity" and "predatory" characters with disability as part of the required reading list in secondary schools. Few educators venture into discussion of these characters and the problematization of disability in such readings (Ware, 2001, 2007).

Faulkner's Benjy Compson in *The Sound and the Fury* (1929), Lennie Small in Steinbeck's *Of Mice and Men* (1937), and Boo Radley in Lee's *To Kill a Mockingbird* (1960) each advance the narrative arc of the novel—yet these particular characters are rarely considered through a disability studies lens. When educators attempt to recall how their teachers broached disability themes in these works, it was often little more than a rudimentary characterization by disability category that served to erase the individual and their humanity (Ware, 2001). How then might we invite students to ask: "Was desire attributed to these characters?" "How might we explore the meaning these characters made of the desires each expressed?" The meaning of desire, or more specifically the "desirability of disability" (Hahn, 1981; 1988), is an obvious first step for educators to consider so that they might enact more realistic engagement with disability throughout the curriculum.

Moving beyond the 'absences-on-disability-and-desire' conversation with teachers, community members, and parents/caregivers will require thoughtful and critical media exposure to provide insights into cultural perceptions about sexuality and disability as it is lived today. We would consider recent films such as: *The Sessions* (Lewin, Hawkes, & Hunt, 2012), *Rust and Bone* (Audidard & Cassinelli, 2012), and *The Scarlet Road* (Scott, 2011) among the media that is readily available. *The Sessions* is based on a short essay by Mark O'Brien (1990), a poet and polio survivor who revisits his youth in Berkeley, California where he won the right to access sexual surrogacy. The film challenges viewers on many levels as it raises issues relative to sexuality and disability that were more freely discussed then than now. *Rust and Bone* raises important questions about disability identity as the female protagonist becomes disabled and new ways of being in the world, including her sexuality, must be re-evaluated. The final film, *The Scarlet Road*, is a documentary set in Australia. It offers a bold glimpse into the world of sexual surrogacy and includes a refreshing perspective from parents who come to realize the contradictions inherent in the path of advancing full inclusion and rights for their children as they move into adulthood. Although it is unlikely these films would ever appear in a secondary curriculum, educators, community members, and parents/caregivers might use the themes of these films to inform their understanding of disability and sexual subjectivity.

Along with the writings of Palacios, Rousso, Finger, Clare, and others, these pieces could help pave the way for explicit connections by parents/caregivers—to their children, and for educators—to the students in their classes. This endeavor will, by design, necessitate a productive partnership between educators and parents/caregivers. Unlike other school-based reform initiatives, it will not be sustained by rhetorical claims to inclusion and the importance of 'community.' This partnership must precede the more critical aspect of turning our attention to the real challenge posed by listening to students, who, similar to the young women in Cowley's data, fully understand the danger of maintaining this silence.

*Linda Ware would like to thank Emily Nusbaum, University or San Francisco, and Abby Ferber, Andrea Herrera, and Heather Albanesi of the Women's and Ethnic Studies Department (WEST) at the University of Colorado, Colorado Springs, for their generous support of her work during her Fall 2013 sabbatical. Our conversations made a lasting marking on my thinking.

REFERENCES

Abbott, D., & Howarth, J. (2007). Still off-limits? Staff views on supporting gay, lesbian, and bisexual people with intellectual disabilities to develop sexual and intimate relationships? *Journal of Applied Research in Intellectual Disabilities, 20*, 116–126.

Artiles, A. J. (2005). Special education's changing identity: Paradoxes and dilemmas in views of culture and space. In L. Katzman, A. G. Gandhi, W. S. Harbour, & J. D. LaRock (Eds.), *Special education for a new century* (pp. 85–120). Cambridge, MA: Harvard Educational Review.

Ashby, C. (2012). Disability studies and inclusive teacher preparation: A socially just path for teacher education. *Research and Practice for Persons with Severe Disabilities, 37*(2), 89–99.

Audidard, J. (Director/Producer), & Cassinelli, M. (Producer). (2012). *Rust and bone* (Motion Picture). France: Why Not Productions.

Aunos, M., & Feldman, M. A. (2002). Attitudes toward sexuality, sterilization and parenting rights of persons with intellectual disabilities. *Journal of Applied Research in Intellectual Disabilities, 15*, 285–296.

Baker, B. (2002). The hunt for disability: The new Eugenics and the normalization of school children. *Teachers College Record, 104*(4), 663–703.

Baglieri, S., Vale, J. W., Connor, D. J., & Gallagher, D. J. (2011). Disability studies in education: The need for a plurality of perspectives on disability. *Remedial and Special Education, 32*(4), 267–278.

Berne, P. (Director). (2013). *Sins Invalid* (Documentary). New Day Films. New York: Blooming Grove.

Biklen, D. (1988). The myth of clinical judgment. *Journal of Social Issues, 44* (1), 127–140.

Biklen, D. (1992). *Schooling without labels: Parents, educators, and inclusive education*. Philadelphia, PA: Temple University Press.

Blatt, B. (1984). *In and out of books: Reviews and other polemics on special education*. Baltimore, MD: University Park Press.

Block, P. (2000). Sexuality, fertility, and danger: Twentieth–century images of women with cognitive disabilities. *Sexuality and Disability, 18*(4), 239–254.

Bogdan, R., & Biklen, S. (2006). *Qualitative research for education: An introduction to theory and methods*. Upper Saddle River, NJ: Allyn and Bacon.

Charlton, J. I. (2000). *Nothing about us without us: Disability oppression and empowerment*. Berkeley, CA: University of California Press.

Chenoweth, L. (1996). Violence and women with disabilities. *Violence Against Women, 2*(4), 391–411.

Colker, R. (2005). *The disability pendulum. The first decade of Americans with Disabilities Act*. New York: New York University Press.

Cowley, D. (2013). *"Being grown": How adolescent girls with disabilities narrative self-determination and transitions* (Unpublished doctoral dissertation). Syracuse, NY: Syracuse University Press.

Cowley, D., Gebb, A., & Guthrie, S. (April 2015). *"They say sex isn't for me": Social justice means students with disabilities accessing sexuality education*. American Educational Research Association (AERA) Annual Meeting, Chicago, IL.

Desjardins, M. (2012). The sexualized body of the child: Parents and the politics of 'voluntary' sterilization on people labeled intellectually disabled. In R. McRuer & A. Mollow (Eds.), *Sex and Disability* (pp. 69–88). Durham, NC: Duke University Press.

Faulkner, W. (1929). *The sound and the fury*. New York, NY: Random House.

Finger, A. (1992). Forbidden fruit. *New Internationalist, 233*, 8–10.

Finger, A. (2012). Introduction. In R. McRuer & A. Mollow (Eds.), *Sex and Disability* (p. 2). Durham, NC: Duke University Press.

Gallagher, D. J., Connor, D. J., & Ferri, B. A. (2014). Beyond the too incessant schism: Special education and the social model of disability. *International Journal of Inclusive Education, 18*, 1120–1142. doi:10.1080/13603116.2013.875599

Garland-Thomson, R. (1996). *Extraordinary bodies: Figuring physical disability in American culture and literature*. New York: Columbia University Press.

Gill, M. (2015). *Already doing it: Intellectual disability and sexual agency*. Minneapolis, University of Minnesota Press.

Gordon, P. A., Tschopp, M. K., & Feldman, D. (2004). Addressing issues of sexuality with adolescents with disabilities. *Child and Adolescent Social Work Journal, 21*, 513–527.

Griffiths, D., & Lunsky, Y. (2000). Changing attitudes towards the nature of socio-sexual assessment and education for persons with developmental disabilities and their caregivers. *Journal of Developmental Disabilities, 7*, 34–49.

Hahn, H. (1981). The social component of sexuality and disability. *Sexuality and Disability, 4*, 220–233.

Hahn, H. (1988). Can disability be beautiful? *Social Policy, 18*, 26–31.

Hehir, T. (2005). *New directions in special education: Eliminating ableism in policy and practice*. Cambridge, MA: Harvard Education Press.

Lee, H. (1960). *To kill a mockingbird*. New York, NY: HarperCollins Publishers.

Lehrer, R. (2012). Golem girl gets lucky. In R. McRuer & A. Mollow (Eds.), *Sex and disability* (pp. 231–255). Durham, NC: Duke University Press.

Leicester, M., & Cooke P. (2002). Rights not restrictions for learning disabled adults: A response to Spiecker and Steutel. *Journal of Moral Education, 31*(2), 181–187.

Lewin, B., Hawkes, J., & Hunt, H. (Producers). (2012). *The sessions* (Motion picture). United States: Fox Searchlight Pictures.

Linton, S. (1998). *Claiming disability*. New York, NY: New York University Press.

Linton, S. (2006). *My body politic: A memoir*. Ann Arbor, MI: University of Michigan Press.

Madison, D. S. (2005). *Critical ethnography*. Thousand Oaks, CA: SAGE.

McRuer, R., & Mollow, A. (Eds.). (2012). *Sex and disability*. Durham, NC: Duke University Press.

NYSACRA. (2007). *New York State Office of Mental Retardation and Developmental Disabilities Regulations* (Part 624). Retrieved from http:www.nysacra.org

O'Brien, M. (1990). On seeing a sex surrogate. *Sun magazine*, issue 174. Retrieved from thesunmagazine.org

Oyler, C. (2011). Teacher preparation for inclusive and critical (special) education. *Teacher Education and Special Education, 34*(3), 201–218.

Parkes, N. (2006). Sexual issues and people with a learning disability. *Learning Disabilities Practice, 9*(3), 32–37.

Rousso, H. (2013). *Don't call me inspirational: A disabled feminist talks back*. Philadelphia, PA: Temple University Press.

Scott, C. (Director). (2011). *Scarlet Road* (Documentary film). Australia: Paradigm Pictures.

Snyder, D., & Mitchell, S. (2006). *Cultural locations of disability*. Chicago, IL: University Press.

Steinbeck, J. (1937). *Of mice and men*. New York, NY: Penguin Books.

Stiker, H. J. (1996). De queleques symbolisations de l'infirmite. *Contraste, 4*, 33–48.

Ware, L. (2001). Writing identity and the other: Dare we do disability studies? *Journal of Teacher Education, 52*(3), 107–123.

Ware, L. (2004). Introduction. In L. Ware (Ed.), *Ideology and the politics of (in)exclusion* (pp. 1–8). New York, NY: Peter Lang.

Ware, L. (2005). Many possible futures, many different directions: Merging critical special education and disability studies. In S. Gabel (Ed.), *Disability studies in education: Readings in theory and method* (pp. 103–124). New York, NY: Peter Lang.

Ware, L. (2007). A look at the way we look at disability. In S. Danforth and S. L. Gabel (Eds.), *Vital questions facing disability studies in education* (pp. 271–287). New York, NY: Peter Lang.

Ware, L. (2013). Special education teacher preparation: Growing disability studies in the absence of resistance. In G. Wilgus (Ed.), *Knowledge, pedagogy, and postmulticulturalism: Shaping the locus of learning in urban teacher education* (pp. 153–176). New York, NY: Palgrave.

Wilkerson, A. (2002). Disability, sex radicalism, and political agency. *National Women's Studies Association Journal, 14*(3), 33–57.

8   When Black Girls Became Pretty: Teacher Biography as Source of Student Transformation

Craig Centrie

At that moment I became freshly aware of a situation to which I had grown inured and oblivious: that in a modern industrial culture, the artists constitute, in fact, an ethnic group, subject to the full "native" treatment. We too are exhibited as touristic curiosities on Monday, extolled as culture on Tuesday, denounced as immoral and unsanitary on Wednesday, reinstated for scientific study Thursday, feasted for some obscurely stylish reason Friday, forgotten Saturday, revisited as picturesque Sunday. We too are misrepresented by professional appreciators and subject to spiritual imperialism, our most sacred efforts are plagiarized for yard goods, our histories are traced, our psyches analyzed, and when everyone has taken pleasure of us in his own fashion, we are driven from our native haunts, our modest dwellings are condemned and replaced by a chromium skyscraper.

(Deren, 1983, p. 7)

On December 7, 2009, Carlene Hatcher Polite, professor, professional dancer, political activist, writer, essayist, historic preservationist, and educator, died of breast cancer at the age of 77 in hospice in a quiet neighborhood in a city where Carlene lived and worked since 1971. She wanted no one to know how sick she had become. On her last day, she passed quietly and comfortably surrounded by her close family.

Generations of students whom she had touched throughout her career as an English professor, both in and out of the classroom, at the local university and in city public schools, mourned then, and continue to be touched by her. She was one of those exceptional teachers who made it her business to educate with compassion and care. Her groundbreaking life and struggles make her a role model to all students, especially African American females.

The life history I present here is a personal narrative, primarily of my memories of a 25-year friendship with Carlene, created for the purpose of documenting the brilliantly creative life of this African American woman. Her work influenced African American literature of the civil rights era. Her literary works, commentaries, and articles initiated a new genre of literature that explored the difficulties of interpersonal black relationships. This was significant because the general position of civil rights leaders of the time was to remain silent on the internal conflicts of the black community. They were concerned the challenges of male/female relationships would dilute the central cause of civil rights.

This narrative is also an example of how the life stories of teachers, community members, and other role models can be used to inspire students to challenge the system. Given the extent of silencing and obstacles in the lives of females, particularly those of color, it is important to excavate, learn from, and celebrate the lives of women who do great things through organizing and resistance. We cannot let those stories be silenced or untold or we too participate in silencing.

The groundbreaking work of feminists such as bell hooks (1989) alerts us to the fact that so much of the official history of the world presented to us focuses on the accomplishments of white males to the near absence of females and other men. Public school curricula by extension reflect this orientation. Despite the considerable contributions of feminist discourse over the last 50 years, there continues to be a palpable absence of female voices, especially those of African Americans and others of color in education. This is most especially true in public schools in urban settings where students from culturally dominated groups compose the majority of the student body, and their teachers are primarily white (Nieto, 2002).

Pierre Bourdieu and Jean-Claude Passeron (1977) explore how schools are primary locations where social reproduction occurs, and they are institutions where symbolic violence is commonplace. The hidden curriculum, and indeed the formal curriculum of schools, perpetuates structures of inequality along racial, gender, and class lines. Policymakers partake in embedded form of symbolic violence, for instance, as they blame poor academic performance on students and their families, rather than on the structured classism and racism of the institution and larger culture (Tosholis, 2012). The structural reality of overcrowded schools and corporate testing regimes have likewise trapped teachers and administrators in settings that are destined to fail (Hall, 2001).

Theorists such as Ladson-Billings (2009) have written on the ways in which schools can be relevant to their students. She asserts that successful teaching of African American children is much less dependent on the race, gender, or ethnicity of teachers than on the willingness of the teacher to work with the unique strengths of the student through culturally relevant means. Still, however, resource allocation is crucial. Other theorists such as Hill-Collins (2009) have further posited that oppression is not merely a matter of a singular marker such as race, but rather it is the intersectionality of race, class, gender, and sexuality which creates multiple layers of oppression. Within these contested spaces, the stories of teachers as sources of inspiration can play a curricular part in making connections with students.

NOTES ON METHODS AND PROCESS

This chapter is presented in storytelling style, a technique regarded as integral to critical race theory in which storytelling/counter storytelling and "naming one's own reality" is used to explore racial oppression (Delgado & Stefancic, 2011). It has been my habit throughout most of my adult life to maintain a diary. My many visits and social engagements, both formal and informal, with Carlene Hatcher Polite always found their way into my personal writing. Carlene was a very knowledgeable, worldly, and witty person whose comments and thoughts I found worth remembering. A visit with Carlene was almost always indelible and inspiring. I am not suggesting she did not experience bad times or that she was not occasionally irritable. It was the artistic side of her personality, the dramatic idiosyncratic part of an accomplished artist, that made each visit worth recounting.

In retrospect, I believe our initial friendship was based on common interests. For me, Carlene was undoubtedly the personification of an artist. I am speculating that she identified in various ways with me as a kindred spirit. I was a photographer and oil painter and was part of the local arts community and university community. I was also raised in the French speaking Antilles and identify as a male of Creole origin. My time spent in Haiti was of particular interest to Carlene, as she was able to discuss her experiences and interests with Afro-Caribbean religions without any explaining.

It was not until after Carlene's death that it occurred to me to write about her for myself as a way to work through the emotions of her passing. Although Carlene was retired from her work as a professor for nine years at the time of her death, it saddened me that the university and her department colleagues did not memorialize her to the extent that they had done for other faculty with a formal service. The chapter presented here is more in keeping with informal reminiscing. I began by locating her daughter and chatting about my friendship with Carlene and all the years that had passed. I then began pulling out all my old diaries to revisit our times together. I contacted many of her friends, colleagues, and family members to crosscheck my memory of dates, locations, and other facts. Because the majority of these individuals lived across the country, and in some cases, abroad, most of the interviews were done over the telephone, and in a few instances through email. During telephone conversations, I kept notes by hand and then typed the information for future triangulation during the analysis and writing stage. With permission, I was occasionally able to tape a telephone communication for more accurate detail. With various individuals who lived locally, it was possible to conduct a more formal interview in person. All interviews were guided by general and open-ended questions to allow the narrator as much freedom as possible to express their feelings and memories. Interviews were initially intended to last no more than 45 minutes. However, in many cases, the subjects enjoyed the experience and the interview did not end until they were ready to end it. All interviewees were knowledgeable of the purpose of the interview beforehand. After brief greetings and general conversation, I only interrupted a narrator's history for points of clarification.

Because many individuals who knew and worked with Carlene are still living and have requested anonymity, contributors to this chapter have been given pseudonyms or are referred to in a few cases as the narrator. The name of the mid-sized northeastern city has been replaced by a fictitious place I call 'Nickel City.' The names of people and some places have also been changed. To complete this storytelling, I have informally and formally interviewed members of her family, personal friends, colleagues, and students who knew Carlene, and were able to fill in parts of Carlene's life about which I only had general or little information. In total, 47 people were interviewed to complete this reminiscence. I also interviewed individuals who did not know Carlene well, but who could provide important context for her life and experiences. What I do not attempt to do is to examine critically her literary work to any great extent or to analyze to any considerable degree how her experiences and life influenced her writing.

Disappointingly, although recognized as a major literary figure in what some critics have called the most important resurgence of black literature since the Harlem Renaissance, I found very little written about Carlene Polite. Her work, however, is listed frequently in bibliographies and reviews of African American literature of the 1960s and 1970s.

Since the publication of Carlene's last book, *Sister X and the Victims of Foul Play* (1975), much of her considerable political work has been over-looked. With dismay, I find her literary work and essays have all but fallen into obscurity. Like many of her friends, I could remember the title of various essays and articles from conversation with Carlene but was unable to find hard copies. Many of her articles appeared in popular and cutting edge magazines during the 1960s. Calls and emails to the editorial offices of those magazines still in existence went unanswered. After several attempts to contact her publisher, I received an email stating everyone who knew her personally had died, and no one currently on staff had any information on Carlene or personal memories to recount.

As I further attempted to research published information on Carlene Hatcher Polite, I was confronted with the surprising lack of information on black female writers generally. Although I believe documenting the works of these important contributors to the American literary experience has improved since the late 1970s, there still are major absences overall. I find this to be a commentary on academia's persistence to focus more attention on males. What follows is merely a beginning of sorts to understand the life of Carlene Hatcher Polite and to provide a context for her experiences from the living memories of those who knew her. I have compared my personal knowledge with those few scholarly commentaries already written about her.

STORY TELLING: REMEMBERING CARLENE
HATCHER POLITE

I met Carlene for the first time in September 1980 at an American Studies
start up party held in the garden of a university professor. Department par-
ties and potluck dinners were commonplace back then. Carlene was just
appointed as the new chair although she only remained chair for fewer than
two months. The politics of higher education, she often said, did not suit
her. She commented frequently that there were many things about academic
life she did not like, but it was the politics of academia she disliked the most.
She was especially dismayed with grading policies. On this fall day in 1980,
students and faculty were eager to meet and talk to her, many for the first
time. For new graduate students such as me, the occasion was filled with
excitement and the usual angst typical for students everywhere. Carlene had
not yet arrived although the party had been in progress for two hours.

Shaped by the civil rights movement, American Studies was one of the
few places at the university where diversity was integral to its mission,
bringing together numerous ethnic and political groups. Initially many of
the programs that comprised American Studies, such as Native American
Studies, Puerto Rican Studies, and Women's Studies, were separate depart-
ments. A shift in conservative university politics downgraded these depart-
ments into programs, perhaps in the hopes of silencing disruptive voices.
However, the effect of placing all of these groups together in one department
created ideas that irritated upper administration. Everyone appeared to be
sharing a common history of marginalization and looked to creating a new
world. It was a time when the memory of civil rights was still fresh, black
was still beautiful, and change still felt possible.

I was sitting in a folding chair talking to two women, one from Chile and
another from Iran. A beautiful black woman dressed in a sort of sophisticated
eclectic style appeared and joined us, but sat several arms-length distant from
the group of us who sat in a circle. The woman from Chile, an artist and
recent refugee from the Pinochet regime and faculty member in Women's
Studies, met Carlene earlier and exclaimed in a rather dramatic voice, "Oh
Carlene! You are finally here. We've been waiting for you!" Our attentions,
of course, immediately switched to the stylish Carlene who introduced herself to us but seemed to me to feel rather tentative, perhaps almost shy.

Our little group had temporarily broken up, but I remained in a circle of
empty chairs and continued to talk to Carlene who now spoke of African
gods and how everyone had a dominant spirit who defined their characters.
Carlene, I had later learned, was a student of African religions, and was
keenly interested in how these religions helped those of the African Dias-
pora survive the inhumanity of the Atlantic slave trade. We had learned in
our brief conversation that we both lived in the same neighborhood, a little
bohemia of sorts. Carlene noted, seemingly out of nowhere, that many Papa
Legbas lived out there. This comment references one of the major gods of
the Voudou pantheon responsible for opening religious ceremonies and the

beginning of all major undertakings. He is represented as a tattered old man in western Afro-diaspora religions. In this context, she is referring to a large number of likely homeless black men who can be seen collecting bottles in the neighborhood. That introductory conversation began what would become a 25-year friendship with Carlene Hatcher Polite, whose experiences, personality, and friendship continues today to influence my life, along with many others who knew her personally. As a teacher, Carlene left an indelible mark on her students.

The following five interview excerpts were conducted with past students of Carlene. They provide a framework for understanding the importance of her impact on students at the university, students who were, in the 1970s and 1980s, regarded by a colleague of Carlene's as non-traditional or the "new demographic." Anika, a student of Carlene's during the late 1970s and now a higher education administrator, stated:

> C.C.:   I understand from the department secretary you were an
>   undergraduate student of Carlene Polite. Can you tell me
>   a little about her teaching style or your experiences with
>   her as a professor?
>
> ANIKA: Well, the university was an intimidating place, I think, for
>   those of us who came from the black community back
>   then. In many ways it still is. We were often the first per-
>   son in our families to attend college, and institutions of
>   higher learning were seriously intimidating places. I know
>   I felt lost. Often I felt, as did many of my friends, that the
>   professors didn't really want us there. I rarely ran into a
>   black face in offices or in the classroom. You know, it was
>   alienating. But I heard about this black woman who was
>   an author and teaching in the English department. A few
>   of my friends and I got her name and we searched for her
>   in the catalogue. What can I say? Professor Polite was
>   amazing! . . . On our first day I thought, wow, it is possible
>   to be black, female, and somebody. She was stylish and
>   smart and encouraging. Every class was an adventure. She
>   encouraged us to stay with it, keep going no matter what
>   and get that degree. Most importantly, she stressed "be
>   yourself and don't make apologies for who you are."

Like Anika, Kamaw, now a freelance videographer and one time "Minister of Information" for the Black Student Union, comments:

> KAMAW: It was the seventies, I heard of Carlene but first met her
>   when she came to meetings of the Black Student Union.
>   She didn't come just to listen and sit in or come there as
>   a big know-it-all professor telling us what to do. Like
>   everyone else I couldn't believe it. She came to act as a

secretary. She came to take notes and type them up for our records. And she did that for years. She came to get involved and to work and do what we were doing. She came in as one of us. She was Carlene Hatcher Polite, a big name in black literature and a Pulitzer Prize nominee, and she came to do work. You couldn't help to be inspired by her and to be encouraged. She was just simply an amazing lady.

Whereas most student interviews were with African American former students, there were white students too who were encouraged and moved by her teaching and lectures.

HOLLY: I first met Carlene in the early 1990s as an undergraduate student taking a black literature course in the American Studies and English Department. Carlene had legions of diehard students who followed her from class to class, and I wanted to see what this was all about. In a giant class with all her fans, I was the white, shy, quiet girl, and new to the authors we were reading: Martin Bernal, Chiekh Anta Diop. In class, Carlene was her genuine self, always alive and on stage, and my classmates and I were enthralled. . . . It was the ways of thinking she presented and the way she listened. Carlene made a point to get to know me and help me feel confident. She helped me realize it was okay and in fact appropriate to study both poetry and education policy, and she confirmed my belief that these things were always wholly connected. Because of her, I ended up in the field of cultural foundations of education.

In the following interview, a student who had taken courses with Carlene and who was encouraged by her to go to graduate school was unaware Carlene had died:

JAMILLA: I'm sorry, you said she passed away? Professor Polite is dead? (Jamilla tries to hold back tears and then reaches for tissues in her purse.) I apologize. I had no idea. Miss Polite, she was really something. Every class was interesting. Each conversation with her was, I don't know, like an epiphany for me. I came to school, I wasn't sure if I could make it or not, you know. I was an EOP (Equal Opportunity Program) student. She was so special. She made me feel like I was somebody. I mean, here you are with this published writer who made waves in the 60's and 70's and who worked with Martin Luther

King and all these names from the Civil Rights Movement that she knew personally and she was talking to me and encouraging me to keep on. . . . I wasn't doing well in school for the first two years, but then I took courses with her and she made me to want to finish. Now, I'm in graduate school, and I credit her with support I needed to keep working. I will never forget her.

Like Jamilla, there were many people, former students of hers and colleagues, who were not aware that Carlene had died, as the university and her department had not made an extensive public statement:

> JOHN: Professor Polite? She passed away? Wow, I had no idea. How come no one knows about this? . . . I took one class with her. It was nearly impossible to get any more because they were all full, sometimes, way in advance. I wanted more classes with her but couldn't get in. She really blew my mind. Just seeing her in class was like, I don't know, like a stage performance with meaning. I feel cheated I didn't get to take more classes with her. But she retired. I can understand that.

All the students I spoke with, like the ones quoted above, viewed Carlene as making them feel special. They say she worked with issues that were relevant to them and viewed each person as an individual. What was also clear from former student interviews is they were not made to feel their lack of comfort in a formal educational institution was a negative, or that their challenges were insurmountable. Rather she was quick to explain the effects of structural sorting and to encourage students to continue their education and move forward. Challenges, in fact, were viewed by Carlene as opportunities.

Student interviews also reveal various aspects of Carlene's personality and teaching style. She involved herself personally in college activities such as offering to be the typist and secretary for a student organization. Faculty involvement in student organizations is often viewed as a mixed blessing by club members. Too often faculty members promote their own interests in such settings. In this case, Carlene may have felt an affinity to the goals of the Black Student Union but did not insert herself as a leader but rather as an equal and working member.

EARLY LIFE

Carlene Hatcher Polite was born in Detroit, Michigan, in 1932 to John and Lillian (Cook) Hatcher. She attended public schools and graduated from Nathan High School in Detroit. Carlene was strongly influenced by her parents. Both parents were important representatives of the United Auto

Workers-Congress of Industrial Workers (UAW-CIO). Her father John was primarily involved in local Detroit politics and the local rights of workers on the floors of the plant. Her mother Lillian was integral to the national and international work of the UAW, acting as its international liaison on civil rights. She often spent a great deal of time in Washington D.C., testifying in front of Congress. In particular, it was the work of Lillian Hatcher that would most shape Carlene's political involvement in the civil rights movement and her life-long interest in human rights. Civil rights officials such as George Meany, president of the UAW, and A. Philip Randolph, a leader in the civil rights movement and labor rights movement, were regular visitors to the Hatcher home. Carlene would describe these visits as spirited and exciting. Lively civil rights planning discussions were some of Carlene's first memories. Visits by high profile civil rights leaders were a constant presence throughout her childhood until she left for New York City.

Before Carlene graduated from high school, she became pregnant at age 17 with her first daughter. Although Carlene would become a teenage mother, this did not discourage her from considering higher education or pursuing her interest in becoming a professional dancer. In fact, she had applied to various prestigious colleges and was accepted into both Sarah Lawrence and New York University. However, contrary to her biography by Frank E. Dobson, Jr. (1999) (in Samuel Nelson's *Contemporary African Writers: A Bio-bibliographical Critical Source Book*), Carlene did not matriculate at Sarah Lawrence College. She did not attend any traditional institution of higher education, having been discouraged with what she later described in a personal communication as "institutional confinements of colleges and universities." In the same biography, Dobson references Carlene as full professor, an academic career elevation her University records do not support.

Although accepted to various colleges and universities, she decided to return to Detroit and marry her daughter's father. There her husband carved out a basic living as an artist/ draftsman. It was during this time when Carlene planned to pursue her interests in the arts. Early in her life, Carlene exhibited talent in various artistic areas including dancing and writing. As a child and teenager she often traded short stories with her cousin, a now internationally recognized writer. However, it was dancing and voice at that time that interested her the most. Carlene, her husband, and their young daughter moved to New York City when Carlene was 19 to pursue a life of their own, as she described it, and be a dancer and maybe "even an opera singer."

Carlene Hatcher Polite spoke very limitedly about her early life in New York City but described it as difficult, with her young husband making a living as an artist/draftsman for the Brooklyn Yards, and she taking various jobs, including working at a large bookstore chain. It was also at this time, in 1949, when she was accepted into The Martha Graham School of Dance, thus beginning her career as a dancer. After a while, Carlene broke off their relationship.

From 1955 to 1959, Carlene pursued her dancing career working in the professional companies of Martha Graham and Alvin Ailey in New York.

Later, when she returned to Detroit, she danced at Vanguard Playhouse and Equity Theater. She performed in many productions and was a featured artist in various performances, including "The King and I," "The Boyfriend," and "Dark of the Moon." As a professional dancer, Carlene met people involved in the performing arts and the cultural community of New York City. These new friendships and acquaintances influenced and inspired the young Carlene, especially her interest in writing.

THE BEGINNINGS OF A LITERARY CAREER

In the early 1950s, Greenwich Village, a neighborhood in lower Manhattan, was still an inexpensive place to live. Described as an artist's haven, it was the center of bohemian life, and during this time the birthplace of the Beat movement (Strenberg, 2007). As her dancing career began to take shape, Carlene met many performers, writers, poets, musicians, and visual artists. Shortly after she moved to Greenwich Village, Carlene met a young, emerging black poet named Allen Polite. He had just returned from the armed services after being stationed in Japan during the Korean War, and the two began a formal relationship. She would later describe meeting him as an important milestone in her life. Carlene began her life with her poet love on Bedford Street in Greenwich Village. It was here too that Carlene would have her second daughter.

Their home, Carlene would describe, was a meeting place where writers and artists from all over New York City would come to eat and chat, including many Greenwich Village luminaries of the times. A now famous writer commented in a personal correspondence:

> When I first visited [my friend] in "the Village" he was living with Carlene on Bedford St. I was immediately in the midst of quite a few young artists who were Allen and Carlene's friends and peers. These included Mercer Cunningham and John Cage and a host of young black painters and writers as well as Zen Buddhist advocates (Harvey Cropper, Vincent Smith, Karl Macbeth, Percy Knight, and Virginia Cox & Co). Carlene was so beautiful; the first sight of her was stunning. She was also the lone black dancer (then) in Mercer Cunningham's company. Their all white Bedford St. apartment had walls covered with books, which they allowed me to peruse and read even while they were away.

Although their list of friends and acquaintances reads like the who's who of avant garde in New York City, many of Carlene's closest friends were those members of the black literati who became critical of the civil rights approach of the NAACP and viewed the movement as in need of more radical politics. Many of their friends were followers of Malcolm X and attended sermons and lectures he gave at his mosque in Harlem. Carlene recounts how she was often criticized for "not being black enough and not having her politics in the right place." Carlene would later comment that she had not gone to New York City to live in Harlem but rather moved there to experience all of its culture and humanity. Similarly, Carlene often felt unsure of her naturally straight hair, as to some this was evidence of her politics of being too white. For Carlene, these comments harkened back to her childhood school days in Detroit when she was teased about her appearance. Her straight hair was a major focus of bullying. During the nearly 25 years I knew Carlene, I never saw her hair. She was always seen with her signature black beret or tied her hair up casually in one of her colorful kerchiefs.

While working at a bookstore, Carlene's fiancé wrote poetry and essays and was a frequent reader at many jazz-poetry cafes around New York City and in private salons. His work was published in *Yungen* and *The London Anthology: Sixes and Sevens*. It was also during this time that Carlene was inspired to return to her old childhood interest in writing poetry, which she also read in jazz poetry cafes and salons around the city.

RETURN TO DETROIT

In early 1960, at age 28, Carlene and her daughters returned home to Detroit because she felt disillusioned with New York City. Her relationship also ended. Shortly after returning, and with the encouragement and contacts of her mother, Carlene became involved in local and national civil rights politics. In his biographical work on her, Dobson (1999) writes:

> In the early 60's, Polite was active in political organizing and the civil rights issues. In 1962 she was elected to the Michigan State Central Committee of the Democratic Party. She coordinated the Detroit Council of Human Rights in the June 1963 Walk for Freedom and the 1963 Freedom Now Rally to protest the Birmingham, Alabama, church bombings. In 1963 she organized the Northern Negro Leadership Conference. (p. 384)

In addition, a family member comments that Carlene was also very much involved in the UAW labor rights movement, participated in the original student sit-ins, was a founding member of a women's rights collectivity, and remembers her being present with her mother in the Detroit city riots. Familiar civil rights faces at their home were such notable icons in the 1960s as Adam Clayton Powel and Rev. C. L. Franklin. Carlene developed close friendships with Carl Stokes, the black mayor of Cleveland (and the first black mayor of any US city) and Coleman Young. Carlene also met with Rev. Martin Luther King on various occasions to discuss civil rights agendas and strategies. Through her political activism, Carlene developed a philosophy of human rights that crossed national boundaries. However, formal organized politics was not a comfortable fit for Carlene. One narrator states: "Although [Carlene] had developed a strong outgoing and outspoken personality, she was not confrontational, and especially didn't like the muckraking that was part of the political process." Carlene often mentioned in personal conversations that she was, in fact, more comfortable with jazz musicians than she ever was with politicians. She also developed a close personal friendship with Berry Gordy, the founder of Motown Records, through whom she would meet the rising stars of soul music.

Although her various roles in politics and civil rights provided her with some income, Carlene also taught modern dance in the Martha Graham technique for Vanguard Playhouse, Equity Theater from 1960 to 1962, and both The Young Women's Christian Association and The Young Men's Christian Association from 1960 to 1963. These part time jobs also provided Carlene with a necessary creative outlet that was likely more in keeping with her personality. During this same period in Detroit, Carlene took on several other odd jobs to supplement her income. In one case, Carlene and her daughters were featured in a car TV commercial whose purpose was to sell their vehicles, but also to promote upscale cars to the new up and coming African American middle class of the post-WWII era.

In late 1963, Carlene accepted a two-week invitation to visit Paris. I spoke with several people who knew who invited Carlene but would not disclose who had invited her. After the visit, she decided to move there for an extended stay. She left, as she would later say, for intellectual freedom and to experience culture.

BECOMING AN EXPATRIATE

In 1964, Carlene and her youngest daughter left New York City on the S.S. France bound for Paris where she would spend the next 8 years of her life. Her oldest daughter remained in Detroit with her mother, as it was agreed that traveling to Europe would not be the best option for a teen who was midway through high school. In Paris, Carlene focused on writing. Several editors encouraged her to write more extensively, a book in particular. She had already written various essays, commentaries, and poems that had been featured in magazines. In 1966, for its first novel, the editor of a new publishing house published *The Flagellants* in French. In 1967, Farrar, Straus, and Giroux published it in English. During the next several years, after a Pulitzer Prize nomination for *The Flagellants*, Carlene received a fellowship from the National Foundation for the Arts and Humanities in 1967 and a Rockefeller Foundation Fellowship in 1968. These awards supported her while she continued to write commentaries and essays on her experiences as an African American in France. Her daughter recalled Carlene would "lock herself up in a room. From the outside I could hear the tap tap tap of the typewriter." However, the 8 years Carlene and her daughter spent in Paris was not all work. Paris during the 1960s was a magnet for African Americans, especially artists. Although Carlene often commented to me and other friends that she went to France to make a separation from her life in the US, it was inevitable that she and other African Americans would miss all things familiar from home.

Carlene and other African Americans who were in Paris during the 1960s gathered in Chez Haynes, a soul food restaurant in the 9th arrondissement. It was opened by Leroy "Roughhouse" Haynes in 1949, and was located at 3 Rue Clauzel, a narrow winding street offering an imposing view of Sacre Coeur above (Dryer, 2010). At Chez Haynes, black visual artists, jazz musicians, writers, and other members of the US expatriate community came to discuss politics, art, and all they missed from home, including southern cooking. During her years in France, Carlene became friends with notable artists, including jazz singer Nina Simone and saxophone artist Charlie Parker. Much of her time was spent in jazz clubs. It was the sounds of jazz, she often remarked, that inspired her writing and the style for which she was noted. Nearly all critics of her work comment that her prose evokes the emotions inherent to jazz (Lee, 2003).

Although Carlene wrote two novels and, since the late 1980s, worked on a third novel, essays, and commentaries, it is *The Flagellants* for which Carlene is most remembered.

The Flagellants was in many ways revolutionary, exploring a topic rarely touched upon by contemporary writers: the tribulations and experiences of black couples. In a news release announcing her death dated December 18, 2009, the university where she had taught describes her writing as follows:

> A lyrical and much-praised protest of the limited gender roles available to African American women and men, it was one of the first works of African American fiction to move beyond the conventions of realism. It garnered major critical attention and distinguished Polite as a member of the first important African American arts movement since the Harlem Renaissance. (Donovan, 2009)

Once, in a conversation with Carlene about her writing, she remarked she had taken "a considerable amount of flack" from the black intellectuals, black men specifically. *The Flagellants* was viewed by many as presenting black men in a bad light. This was a book, however, that Carlene felt she had to write. In later conversations, she commented that much of *The Flagellants* was based on her relationship(s). These strong females in Carlene's family taught her that women must have an identity and life separate from the men in their lives and should rely on themselves for self-worth and financial wellbeing.

Carlene recounted the many limitations, indignities, and humiliations put upon male family members and friends. In a racist society, black males are routinely subjected to the inability to find suitable employment or any work, thereby taking away one of the most basic expectations of masculinity to be the provider and the protector. Faced with these realities, black women struggle to provide for and protect themselves, their children, and often the men in their lives. Within the African American family, this dichotomy between what is expected and what is real becomes a typical and routine contradiction. Much of the verbal and physical violence she remembers in her life in Greenwich Village in the 1950s was portrayed in *The Flagellants* between the characters Ideal and Jimson. To a certain extent, when revisiting my conversations with Carlene, I believe writing *The Flagellants* was necessary to put into perspective her life experiences.

Unfortunately, I also believe the inner existential conversations of being both black and female, which Carlene also explored in fiction in the 1960s and 1970s, would continue to haunt her. This would arguably play out in her work as a professor during the second half of her life. After writing *The Flagellants*, Carlene became fascinated by the biography of Josephine Baker. Baker's early years became a basis for the character of Abyssinia, the protagonist in her second novel, *Sister X and the Victims of Foul Play (1975)*.

The tremendous cultural experiences, artistic offerings, and cosmopolitan atmosphere of Paris inspired Carlene in areas of art and historic conservation. It also provided Carlene with a vantage point to view the constructs of race, class, and sexism from a unique perspective. Carlene would later comment that her outsider status provided a lens to view these topics without the usual accompaniment of emotional self-involvement. What I understood this to mean is that while in France there appeared to be mitigated racism toward African Americans, but this was just a facade. France, of course, had for centuries been involved in the exploitation of the African continent and also parts of the Caribbean, South East Asia, and many other areas in the world. Ingrained institutional and structural racism certainly occurred in France, and as Carlene would comment, it was very similar to the experiences of African Americans in the US. This more complex understanding of the overall nature of racism in Paris would later come into play in her novel *Sister X*.

Exploring these subjects in unique ways made her a popular speaker and essayist. Carlene's family recalls she was often invited to the US Embassy as a guest of Sargent Shriver, the ambassador to France. By 1969, Carlene began to miss her life in the states. She was also concerned, as she did not want her daughter to grow up to be what she described as a "black French girl." I understand this comment to mean she wanted her daughter to be fully socialized in African American culture and history.

In the same conversation, Carlene told the following story about what helped her decide to move back to the US. Carlene knew of an African American man who had lived in Paris for a long time and had absorbed what she described as "French sensibilities." One day, this man heard a loud scuffle on the streets involving a European woman and a North African man. The noise caused passersby and the police to be involved. Like the police, The African American man immediately assumed the North African had done something terrible to the French woman. In fact, it was later found the French woman had tried to pickpocket the man. It was a moment of self-realization for the African American man, who immediately understood he had engaged in racist assumptions in concluding that the North African was the "dangerous other." France as a country free of racism was an illusion. During the last two years in France, she met the chair of an English Department at a university in a northeastern city in the US. He had been passing through the city. After various discussions and negotiations and with the advice of her publishers, in 1971, she accepted a position as an associate professor at that university. Her later tenure was a separate advancement.

MAKING NICKEL CITY A PERMANENT HOME

The English Department at the University at Nickel City (UNC) during the 1960s and most of the 1970s was considered to be one of the most innovative, garnering it the nickname the Berkeley of the East. With an emphasis on writing, poetry, and increasingly criticism, the roster of its faculty was a litany of stars in the literary world, and included Robert Creely, Irving Feldman, and Leslie Fiedler. The English Department was known nationally then as "the hot center, and on the cutting edge" (Jackson, 1999). At the time, the dean gave the chair of the English department a blank check to get faculty who were the best and the brightest. By 1970, the field of English in general was experiencing a paradigm shift. There was an increasing interest in the voices of African Americans and others seldom heard and read.

In 1963, UNC was transitioning from a private university to become part of the State University system. The state government was increasingly requiring the hiring of minorities in its institutions of higher education. As one faculty member from this time reflects:

> With the start of the 70s, minorities, African Americans in particular, were being hired in faculty positions for the first time. But it wasn't easy for these first generation black professors. I remember when Carlene Hatcher Polite was hired. The students were really excited to learn she was coming to join the faculty, and I'm sure that when a position opened at that time, the higher ups, maybe quietly, demanded that it be filled by a black faculty member. Carlene covered two major areas: She was black and she was a woman.

In the fall of 1971, Carlene Hatcher Polite had become the first full time black faculty member hired at the rank of Associate Professor in the English Department.

On the suggestion of UNC staff, Carlene rented a large and elegant house on Southampton in one of Nickel City's most fashionable neighborhoods. There, Carlene and her youngest daughter lived happily while she adjusted to a new life as a faculty member. Carlene often held literary salons in her home where local writers, actors, and artists gathered for food and listened to poetry or excerpts of someone's soon-to-be published novel. Friends and artists alike came to meet one another. In one conversation, I asked if Carlene was recreating in Nickel City the types of experiences she had in New York City or in Paris at Chez Haynes. I was quickly corrected and informed, "Carlene was not recreating anything but continued the life she always lived no matter where she lived it." She was continuing her journey. Professor Johnson, director and playwright, reminisces:

> Carlene was the consummate artist who reminded me of Abby Lincoln, same style, same dress, and of course June Jordan. To watch her was like watching poetry in motion. Carlene was part of the Detroit artist's movement. . . . She was one of the best things that happened in UNC's English Department. I remember once talking to her about a film documenting the life of Charlie Parker. You know she knew Parker quite well. She [Carlene] felt they had done Charlie wrong [in the film], misrepresented him and then [she] made a very deep comment, that she saw herself as a child of Be-Bop . . . and that all of us who were born during this period were the children of Be-Bop, that it defined who we were, who we are. I thought about that a long time and think she was right.

Carlene's second daughter, now a teenager, was registered at the local African American Cultural Center where she learned African dance and interacted with other African American children her age. Carlene often commented that she wanted to ensure her daughter did not become estranged from her heritage. Carlene sought out the local black community and became a regular at Montgomery's, a once upscale, black-owned restaurant that catered to the tastes of famous black performers who came to Nickel City but did not readily eat at the same places they performed. She went to hear jazz at the Colored Musician's Club on The Grand and the local Cotton Club, places where the most famous of blues and jazz artists came to enjoy themselves after performing in white night clubs.

Her first experiences at the university were very positive. University classrooms were beginning to have a noticeable black student presence. The Black Student Union and other newly formed university organizations of color were excited to have such an important writer on the English Department's full time faculty. Shortly after her arrival in Nickel City, her longtime friend and publisher began to encourage her to write her second novel. He firmly believed Carlene was a very talented and special writer with much more to say. He explained to Carlene that it was important for her to continue to produce regularly. She found, however, personal creativity to be difficult while teaching and being a mother. She finally relented in 1974, and had her publisher arrange a hotel room in New York City. In six weeks, Carlene wrote her second novel, *Sister X and the Victims of Foul Play*.

In this novel, Carlene again draws heavily from her personal experiences and creates a character, Arista Polo, a dancer, who performed around the world and who from the beginning of the novel, is dead. Arista, refusing to dance nude, is fired, and while collecting her final paycheck, dies after falling off the stage. Her death is suspicious and raises many questions. Could Ann White from Birmingham, Alabama, and who now dances in Arista's place in black face, have pushed her? Arista's experiences are woven into a series of narrations by Abyssinia, the protagonist or voice that is recounting the story. Abyssinia suggests that black people die from CCC, a constellation of racist experiences that begin with the letter C—such as chain gangs and cotton fields—experiences filled with an historic legacy of killing black people.

Carlene once mentioned she left Detroit for New York City in the hopes of training as an opera singer. Shortly after arriving, she was told by a gatekeeper that "black girls don't become opera singers." It was not, as she explained, whether she had the vocal abilities to pursue this dream, but rather the limitations placed on African Americans and the countless destroyed dreams that devastates the spirit of the individual and the black community as a whole. This crushing comment deeply affected Carlene and become the fundamental premise upon which *Sister X and the Victims of Foul Play* is based. Whereas a list of Carlene's accomplishments suggests a very successful, and as one interviewee stated, "a rather charmed life," this would not accurately portray her internal struggles and experiences with racism and painful relationships as explored in her two novels. A prominent writer and activist who knew Carlene personally explained, "It's not the facts that tell [Carlene Hatcher Polite's] story; it's the context that is the story."

For the next several years, the accomplishment of completing a second novel was very satisfying for Carlene. She was often invited to read at literary events locally and in New York City. The now famous "Literary Center of Nickel City" had her discuss her works and career and contracted her along with other writers to create a now misplaced collection of poems and essays entitled *Yes, Dear Reader* (1978). Her classes at the university were filled to capacity.

By 1980, however, the novelty of teaching at a large academic institution began to wane. Carlene, always very private and wanting to keep her personal life separate from her professional life, had declined invitations to faculty gatherings so often she was eventually rarely invited to join. While interviewing people for this chapter, I contacted individuals from her department who stated they never met her or did not know anything about her. Carlene often complained the English Department consistently required her to teach introductory level courses while assigning younger recent hires

more interesting topic specific courses. She was often asked to teach in undesirable time periods and always refused. When Carlene was granted tenure,
several of her colleagues made it known they felt she did not deserve it and
suggested the only reason she received tenure was because she was pretty.
This was a sentiment Carlene greatly resented, reminding her of comments
directed to her earlier that black girls do not become opera singers. In one
conversation with me, she remarked that the tenure comment was demean-
ing, and was a refusal to recognize her talent as a writer. As she questioned
out loud, "And when did black girls become pretty, anyway?"

Carlene made it clear she did not agree with much of academic culture
and did not hesitate to make her opinions known. Over the decade, she felt
increasingly alienated from her department and colleagues. The isolation
Carlene experienced at the university was not unique. To explore this point
further, I interviewed various African American academics at the same institution about such issues who taught during the time she did. The responses
I received are a testament to the difficulties African American faculty experienced in the 1960s and 1970s, difficulties which continue today. Dr. Hamp-
ton, a specialist in English, reflects:

> It was very difficult in those days. As all these once private schools
> became part of the state system, departments were being urged to make
> minority hires but individual white faculty were not open to the idea,
> not comfortable with black faculty. We had to work so much harder
> than our white colleagues, having to be experts in all aspects because
> we were given anything and everything to teach. If we didn't, there was
> a fear that we would be viewed as having no talent and only hired for
> being minorities. We didn't have black colleagues to support us because
> we were so few.

This sentiment was held by nearly every female and male African American
faculty member I interviewed. One narrator who did not want to be identified specifically stated:

> It (the English department) had made a shift from writing to criticism.
> This shift in focus made things more difficult for Carlene Polite. She was
> a success as a creative writer, not a critic of dead white men. She didn't
> have a Ph.D. and as far as I know, never attended college or even had a
> bachelor's degree. The fact that she was hired would have pissed off any
> number of the men up there. On top of that, English was an old boys
> club. If you weren't one of them, you just didn't count.

This final comment is supported by an article published in a local arts journal, *The Nickel City Beat*. In this article, the author explores the halcyon
days of (Nickel City's) English Department, naming a long list of important writers of the 1960s and 1970s. Nearly all are white and men, and

Carlene Hatcher Polite is never mentioned although she was hired in 1971. I contacted the author of the piece and asked about the omission of Carlene. He remarked that he did not know her very well, and although she was often invited to their home for gatherings, she never accepted his invitation. An African American author and educator speaking on Carlene's experiences said:

> I certainly knew Carlene and was invited to her home on various occasions, but sadly never got to know her very well. I do know she was very dissatisfied with her experiences at (the university) and felt she wasn't liked by her colleagues. When I met her she had become very cynical of her experiences. . . . For many people she was an enigma. Carlene was the type of black person that whites can't wrap their minds around. She was a successful writer and what I remember was very independent, private, and most of all very bohemian. This is hard for whites to understand that a black woman could be successful and independent. When whites can't figure you out it pisses them off. She was still a black person dealing with an institution racially. She was a black academic working in a department with a white aesthetic. For Carlene this created a conflict and a struggle. She was the type of black they couldn't manage. In the end it's sad that after 30 years of service she wasn't recognized.

When Carlene was invited to speak or present excerpts of her work, she often invited me to come along, sometimes to introduce her and other times just for the support. By the 1990s, I recognized the invitations to speak and present her work came less frequently. Carlene understood it was time to write another novel.

Her longtime friend and publisher continued to invite her to New York City and encouraged her to write another novel but it never was completed. During the 1990s, Carlene became increasingly interested in local black history, especially the history of the Cotton Club, a favorite place of Carlene's and one that hosted several of her readings. By the mid-1990s, the club, now managed by the second husband of its founder, became rather neglected and shabby. The owner, now in his late seventies and in ill health, began to sell many of its historic contents. Carlene purchased several pieces of furniture, one of which was a dressing table with a huge round mirror. Carlene, long interested in history and art conservation, intended to have the dresser completely restored. She also began a campaign to have the club designated as a city historic landmark.

Several times Carlene and I sat in front of the dresser while she mused about the stories the mirror could tell if it could speak. The mirror fascinated Carlene and became the inspiration for her third novel, which was never completed. Although I can no longer remember the exact plot, the inspiration for the novel was Maya Deren's (1983) *Divine Horsemen, The Living Gods of Haiti*. Carlene would talk about the "magical mirror" on the dressing table. The mirror as she described it was entwined with the cosmic metaphor of Haitian divine mythology, in which the souls of the dead reside on the other side of the mirror's reflection, and they began to sink to the abyss of the netherworld until recalled by the living. This, Carlene thought to be a perfect beginning for a novel. She would recall the memories and the souls of the dormant spirits of the many black singers, actors, and musicians who sat in front of this mirror. She would ask them to tell their stories.

CONCLUSION

Regrettably, this was the last long conversation I had with Carlene. We were in touch briefly several times over the remaining years of her life. Carlene had moved on after she retired. Through a personal communication with a friend in January 2010, I was told Carlene had passed away and had lived in a suburb nearby for the past 7 years. She also had gotten married. I was shocked of course. When I had not heard from her, I assumed she was on various trips around the world, as she had often talked about. She wanted to spend time in an ashram in India, travel the Silk Road, revisit Paris, and see the pyramids of Egypt.

In 2012, Carlene's daughter contacted me. She had still not cleaned out her mother's apartment. Carlene continued to maintain her apartment even after she married, I was told, "just in case she had to split." Three years after her passing, it is still much the way she kept it. It was impossible to throw anything out before examining it closely. A first edition book might be signed with a personal message from the author. A scrap of paper might contain a plot for a new book. There are heaps of records, papers, and files that need to be gone over. According to her daughter, "You can't just grab a stack of newspapers or old student papers because when you look carefully, a personal snapshot of Martin Luther King or Charlie Parker is hidden between them." Sometimes, too, a manuscript for something in progress turns up. In my mind I can see her beautiful Victorian mansion apartment, high up several flights of stairs, its stately ballroom her living room, filled with memorabilia of her life.

I miss my friend Carlene. I miss the inspiration, the drama, the wicked sense of humor, and the magic she could bring to every event big and small. Sometimes, when I pass a mirror, I imagine I catch sight of a shadow. I wonder if it could be her reminding me of the message her life gave, that anyone can be anything if they want. You only have to believe in yourself.

REFERENCES

Bourdieu, P., & Passseron, J. C. (1977). *Reproduction in education, society, and culture*. London: Sage Publications.

Delgado, R., & Stefancic, J. (2011). *Critical race theory: An introduction.* New York: New York University Press.

Deren, M. (1983). *The divine horsemen: The living gods of Haiti.* New Paltz: McPherson

Dobson, F. in Nelson, S. E. (1999). *Contemporary African American Novelists: A bio-bibliographical source book.* Westport, CT: Greenwood Press.

Donovan, P. (2009). *Carlene Hatcher Polite: A leading light of the 1960's black arts movement.* Retrieved from http://www.buffalo.edu

Dryer, E. (2010, July 25). *Chez Haynes: Let's not forget this soul food restaurant in the Harlem of Paris.* Pittsburg Post-Gazette. Retrieved from http://www.post-gazette.com

Hall, J. (2001). *Canal town youth: Community organization and adolescent identity.* New York: State University of New York Press.

Hill-Collins, P. (2009). *Black feminist thought: Knowledge, consciousness, and the politics of empowerment.* New York: Routledge.

hooks, b. (2000). *Feminist theory: From margin to center.* Cambridge, MA: South End Press.

Jackson, B. (1999, February 26). Buffalo English: Literary Glory Days at U.B. *Buffalo Beat.* Retrieved from http://acsu.buffalo.edu

Ladson-Billings, G. (2009). *The dreamkeepers: Successful teachers of African American children.* San Francisco, CA: Teachers College Press.

Lee, A. (2003). *Multi-cultural American literature: Comparative Black, Native, Latino/a and Asian American writers.* Jackson, MS: University of Mississippi.

Nieto, S. (2002). *Language, culture, and teaching: Critical perspectives for a new century.* Mahwah, NJ: Erlbaum.

Noddings, N. (1989). *Women and evil.* Berkley: University of California Press.

Polite, C. H. (1967). *The Flagellants.* New York: Farrar, Straus, & Giroux.

Polite, C. H. (1975). *Sister X and the victims of foul play.* New York: Farrar, Straus, &Giroux.

Polite, C. H. (1978). *From sister X and the victims of foul play.* Buffalo, NY: Just Buffalo.

Sternberg, A. (2007). Embers of gentrification. *New York Magazine, 11*(12). http://nymag.com/news/features/40648/

Toshalis, E. (2012). The rhetoric of care: Preservice teacher discourses that depoliticize, deflect, and deceive. *Urban Review, 3*(1), 81–87.

9 Stop the Potlucks

Julia Hall

Females continue to be victimized in evolving ways as an integral feature of capitalist relations. Why have so many critical educators, sociologists, feminists, and policymakers turned their attention away from the reality of violence against girls, seeing the issue as already addressed in prior decades? If it is acknowledged, why is there a tendency to categorize it as just another example of the generic, decontextualized, depoliticized, and watered down concept of 'bullying?' To focus on 'bullying' is to empty out histories of racialized, gendered, sexualized, and class-based violence that manifest in ways that are structural, hegemonic, punitive, and personal (Collins, 2008; Rubin, 1976). It also ignores the cumulative nature of violence, involving compounding and overlapping strands experienced from many sources at the same time. When gender is thought about today in terms of schooling, it is more likely in relation to whether female or male students are gaining or losing an 'edge.' Instead of pitting students against each other—with girls and STEM or the 'boy turn' or the 'boy problem' (experienced by privileged young males) (Brooks, 2012; Pomerantz, Raby, & Stefanik, 2013)—argued is that young people must be encouraged to come together across divisions and seek out their commonality, their creativity, and themselves. Students desperately need public spaces in which to find their collective, critical voices.

Foregrounding this investigation is the broader theoretical contention that in post-Fordist production regimes, neoliberalism needs gender in evolving ways. In this context, the forged qualities of 'feminine' identity—characteristics such as flexibility, creativity, the ability to listen, attentiveness, and attention to detail—are increasingly the valorized attributes of the female *and* male identity as worker, consumer, and entrepreneur (McRobbie, 2010, 2014). The economy today is bound up in these elaborations. Labor, in other words, is becoming feminized. In answering the call to work, as importantly asserted by Goodman (2013), all must be flexible.

Whereas neoliberalism needs gender, in maximizing profit it divides it along lines of the colonial white and the 'Other.' In this sense, 'feminine' traits such as flexibility, creativity, the ability to listen, attentiveness, and attention to detail are part of the 'biological' white ideal. In spite of profuse resistance across groups, capital also continues to misread females from culturally dominated groups as naturalistic—as unwieldy, highly physical, hypersexual, and inattentive. These women require immense 'correction.' This justifies ways in which capital has positioned such females as pliable for exploitation. History shows the labor demands made by capital from women from such groups has been characterized by painful flexibility, compressed labor, and the forced suppression of emotions. Today females continue to face a concentrated world of violence and punishment so more privileged females and their daughters can 'lean in.' The impact of such postcolonial terrains of production on the lives of school age females in cities is of significant concern, especially because feminism as a movement has splintered apart with weakened strands involved in other issues.

In order to envision a future for females and indeed everyone that is not defined by violence, it is worth reflecting on what can be learned from past feminist movements. In terms of organizing, while well intended, white women at times used their privilege to define issues and actions in the name of 'sisterhood.' Although many wanted to organize to disrupt the centrality of violent capitalist relations, those more privileged women were often unable to recognize their reified status and propensity to speak for others. Some were unaware of the contradictions in their ability to attend a consciousness raising session because they employed a domestic worker to care for their children, cook, and clean their homes. As capitalist relations have historically rendered so many females invisible, some white feminists were now doing the same thing. Numerous more privileged white women failed to realize in a sustained way just as all females have been defined according to economic ends, this has been experienced hierarchically. For example, African American girls and women still had to endure the same old and controlling images of 'mammie,' 'welfare cheat,' 'hypersexual,' and 'reproductively reckless.' Such images persist in legitimizing the exploitation of girls and women from all marginalized groups, along with the low wages of females in general. At the same time, they maintain the relative advantaging of white womanhood (Collins, 2008). This disconnect ultimately stymied the development of collectivity across groups. For several decades, feminism as a movement broke off into important debates on identity and poststructuralism. But during this time period, neoliberalism washed across the landscape. Neoliberalism as a set of ideological positions fostered deep divisions among females as part of the larger strategy to divest all potentially challenging social movements of power. This constitutes discrediting from outside but also from within by creating factions.

Fueled by economic developments that began on the ground in the 1970s as global policies (e.g., IMF/World Bank debt, privatizing water), in the 1980s, Thatcher-Reagan drew widespread support at home for an anti-government/racialized gender stance. State regulation was now seen as the result of market weakness, or 'feminine.' As a result, swift and decisive action was ushered in. For example, transportation was deregulated, unions were undermined, and teachers were blamed for being 'soft,' thereby leading to loss of industry and jobs and the rise in inflation. Schools and teachers were seen as ineffective and a significant reason for the undermining of employment. Mired in its weaknesses, feminism and other social movements have not had success in disrupting uses of colonial racialized gender as a form of productivity, for instance, in the form of the 'nanny state.' In this image, government is seen as the feminine 'Other'—large, lazy, wasteful, weak, and always ready for a hand out. It must be replaced with a white, male, corporate-efficient version of governance.

The decade of the 1990s was especially devastating for the obliteration of the 'weak and feminine' social contract via slash and burn policies targeted toward specific class and race groups. During this era, President Clinton (and Blair in the UK) 'reinvented government.' This meant shrinking its regulatory functions. Aided by the World Trade Organization (WTO) rulings, corporate power rapidly increased. The government workforce itself was lacerated by hundreds of thousands. This was a disproportionate assault on especially females from culturally dominated groups, as such jobs were one place of employment that represented more equitable hiring practices. Again, due to the severe lack of opportunities for education and employment afforded their male counterparts, these females were more likely than white women to be supporting an entire family on that single salary. This, along with the gutting of social policy, was especially devastating.

As discussed, the 1996 Personal Responsibility and Work Opportunity Reconciliation Act was punitively directed toward single mothers and caretakers of children. Efforts to control sexuality and the reproductive rights of these women is embedded in the reform in the guise of the 'capped child' clause and the ticking time clock of the limited benefits (Hays, 2003; Wacquant, 2009). The Kennedy-Kassenbaum Fighting Fraud and Waste in Medicare Act was signed that same year (Laws & Regulations, 2014). The intended goal of this act was to coordinate with the Department of Justice to fight fraud, hence implying cheating was so widespread among those who were impoverished it required intervention by the criminal justice system. Federal prosecutors and FBI agents were hired to fight these transgressions, convict, and save billions. Such pieces of legislation presuppose those who are poor and attempt to avail themselves of assistance—mostly women and children—are slothful, characterless criminals who work the system and require sanctioning. The more recent cutting of $40 billion to a food stamp program is yet another example of hyper-masculine state violence directed toward raced and classed populations of children.

Survival for many families today depends on adults working long hours at several minimum wage jobs. It is increasingly difficult for parents and caretakers to turn to the previous generation for help with childcare. In 2000, President Clinton signed the Senior Citizen's Freedom to Work Act into law (Laws & Regulations, 2014). This law eliminates earning requirement limits for people older than the normal retirement age. Instead of calculating social security based on inflation, senior citizens are 'freed' by being thrown back on themselves for survival. Having to take on paid labor in their later years and also often helping watch energetic grandchildren, these women continue to experience the reality of compressed labor, suppressed emotion, and exhaustion. This seems a script many females cannot shake. Even when age and health demand one slows down, many women have no choice but to continue on. While privileged females may plan retirement around the desire to relax, travel, and enjoy family, less resourced women of the same age are their cleaning ladies, dry cleaning attendants, and cashiers. They then go home to help take care of grandchildren.

As long as there is no organized constituency focused on disrupting the violent ways capital produces gender, this brutality and despair will continue. Instead of seeking out our commonality, in the current culture, we are told society should mimic the values of the survival of the fittest. Therefore, produced versions of femininity which benefit capital persist. In this space we are told the only role of citizenship is consumerism. We are led to believe the social contract is a pathology and we are responsible for only ourselves. Employment, if you are worthy enough to get it, is low wage and compressed. The punishments for being unemployed are punitive and painful and this is inflicted on adults and children alike. With school controlled by market interests, as seen in this volume, young people have little way of understanding democracy outside capitalism.

Other ways of thinking are seriously needed. Feminism and other social movements must be centrally involved in fostering such conversations. On the path forward, those who are privileged must think through how they have historically benefited from the denigration of females and males from culturally dominated groups. By groups engaging with others and all we have in common, a radical vision outside fractured voices and individual causes can be imagined. The production of violent, classed, and racialized gender in all its forms must be fully shut down. Linked to this process, in many ways cities are hopeful places. Although neoliberalism is a global force, successful policy construction and implementation is also influenced by local forces and forms (Ball, 2012; Ball, Macguire, & Braun, 2012; Lipman, 2011). With their concentrations and diverse mixes of people, importantly, cities are locations where widespread contestations and critical ideas emerge. Urban areas are, therefore, important spaces for envisioning something above and beyond the violent economy that inscribes the lives of females and everyone (Leitner, Sheppard, Sziarto, & Maringanti, 2007; Lipman, 2011).

REFERENCES

Ball, S. (2012). *Global education inc.: New policy networks and the neo-liberal imaginary*. New York: Routledge.

Ball, S., Macguire, M., & Braun, A. (2012). *How schools do policy: Policy enactments in secondary schools*. New York: Routledge.

Brooks, D. (2012, July 5). Honor code. *The New York Times*. Retrieved from http://www.nytimes.com/2012/07/06/opinion/honor-code.htm

Collins, P. H. (1990/2008). *Black feminist thought: Knowledge, consciousness, and the politics of empowerment*. New York: Routledge.

Goodman, R. (2013). *Gender work: Feminism after neoliberalism*. New York: Palgrave Macmillan.

Hays, S. (2003). *Flat broke with children: Women in the age of welfare reform*. New York: Oxford University Press.

Laws & Regulations. (2014). GPO U.S. Government Publishing Office, Public and Private Laws. Retrieved from http://www.usa.gov/Topics/Reference-Shelf/Laws.shtml

Leitner, H., Sheppard, E., Sziarto, K., & Masringanti, A. (2007). Contesting urban futures: Decentering neoliberalism. In H. Leitner, J. Peck, E. Sheppard (Eds.), *Contesting neoliberalism: Urban frontiers* (pp. 1–25). New York: Guilford Press.

Lipman, P. (2011). *The new political economy of urban education: Neoliberalism, race, and the right to the city*. New York: Routledge.

McRobbie, A. (2010). Reflections on feminism, immaterial labour and the post-fordist regime. *New Formations, 70*, 60–76.

McRobbie, A. (2014). *Be creative: Making a living in the new culture industries*. London: Polity.

Pomerantz, S., Raby, R., & Stefanik, A. (2013). Girls run the world? Caught between sexism and postfeminism in school. *Gender & Society, 27*(2), 185–207.

Rubin, L. (1976). *Worlds of pain: Life in the working-class family*. New York: Basic Books.

Wacquant, L. (2009). *Punishing the poor: The neoliberal government of social insecurity*. London: Duke University Press.

Contributors

Virginia A. Batchelor is Professor of Education at Medaille College in Buffalo, New York. In her work she considers creativity, health, and social issues regarding women and girls. More recently, her research centers on human sex trafficking and youth. She is publishing a book for children that infuses history and social issues.

Linda Burton is Dean of Social Sciences and James B. Duke Professor of Sociology at Duke University. Her work is conceptually grounded in life course, developmental, and ecological perspectives and she focuses on three themes concerning the lives of the poorest urban, small town, and rural families: (1) intergenerational family structures, processes, and role transitions; (2) the meaning of context and place in the daily lives of families; and, (3) childhood adultification and the accelerated life course. She was one of six principal investigators involved in the multisite, multi-method collaborative study of the impact of welfare reform on families and children (*Welfare, Children, and Families: A Three-City Study*).

Craig Centrie is Associate Professor in the School of Education at Medaille College. In his research, he investigates settlement issues and identity formation among students who are immigrants and refugees. His book *The Identity Formation of Immigrant Youth in an American High School* is an exploration of the life experiences of newly arrived Vietnamese students to cities in the US. Centrie is also one of the founders and director of El Museo Gallery, Western New York's only visual arts organization dedicated to the exhibition of artists of color.

Danielle Cowley is Assistant Professor in the Department of Special Education at the University of Northern Iowa. She teaches courses in the areas of behavioral supports, inclusive education, differentiated instruction, and transitions. Her research interests include disability and adolescent girlhood, culturally responsive transition planning, and inclusive school reform. She has published in various journals.

Raymond D. Garrett-Peters is a Sociology Instructor at Duke University.

Julia Hall is Professor of Education Policy at D'Youville College. In her research she considers the school and community experiences of youth who have been economically and culturally marginalized in cities in the context of a rapidly changing economy. She is likewise focused on gendered violence and female students. Her books include *Canal Town Youth: Community Organization and the Development of Adolescent Identity*, *Underprivileged Schoolchildren and the Assault on Dignity: Policy Challenges and Resistance*, and *Children's Human Rights and Public Schools in the United States*.

Craig Haney is Professor of Psychology at the University of California, Santa Cruz. He has won numerous academic honors and awards for distinguished teaching, research, and contributions to constitutional rights. One of the principal researchers on the highly publicized 'Stanford Prison Experiment' in 1971, he has been studying the psychological effects of living and working in actual prison environments since then. Professor Haney has published over 150 journal articles and book chapters on crime, prison, and justice-related topics. He has also written two widely praised books on criminal justice reform, including *Death by Design: Capital Punishment as a Social Psychological System* and *Reforming Punishment: Psychological Limits to the Pains of Imprisonment*.

Ruby Hernandez is a graduate student in the Social Psychology Doctoral Program at the University of California, Santa Cruz. Her research interests include the intersectional and psychological experiences of marginalized communities as shaped through education. She has presented her research at the *National Association for Chicana and Chicano Studies, The Society for the Study of Gloria Anzaldúa*, and *the Society for the Psychological Study of Social Issues*.

Aída Hurtado is Luis Leal Endowed Professor and faculty member in the department of Chicana and Chicano Studies at the University of California, Santa Barbara. She is past chair of the National Association for Chicana/Chicano Studies, Past President of the American Psychology Association's Division 35 (Society for the Psychology of Women) Section III (Issues of Hispanic Women/Latinas), and Chair Elect of MALCS (Mujeres Activas en Letras y Cambio Social-Women Active in Letters and Social Change). She centers her research on intersectional theory, educational achievement, and media representations of race and gender. Her books include *The Color of Privilege: Three Blasphemies on Race and Feminism*; *Voicing Chicana Feminisms: Young Women Speak Out on Sexuality and Identity*; *Chicana/o Identity in a Changing U.S.*

Society, and; *Invisible No More: Understanding the Disenfranchisement of Latino Men and Boys.*

Illana R. Lane is Head of the Division of Education at Medaille College. Her research interests include issues regarding, race, class, gender and children in P-12 schools. Dr. Lane is active in multiple organizations. She is the President of the New York State Association of Educators and serves on the Amherst Central School Board. She is also a member of the Jack and Jill organization.

Alexander J. Means is Assistant Professor in the Department of Social and Psychological Foundations of Education at SUNY Buffalo State. He is the author of *Schooling in the Age of Austerity: Urban Education and the Struggle for Democratic Life* and *Toward a New Common School Movement* with Noah De Lissovoy and Kenneth Saltman.

Lindsay Palmer is Assistant Professor of Global Media Ethics in the School of Journalism and Mass Communication at the University of Wisconsin-Madison. Her work has appeared in the peer-reviewed journals *Genders, Feminist Review, Television and New Media*, and *Continuum*, as well as in various edited collections. Before becoming an academic, Palmer worked as a television news writer and producer in Colorado Springs and San Diego.

Diane Purvin is an independent policy and evaluation research consultant at CT Policy Research in the greater New York City area.

Linda Ware is Associate Professor in the Ella Cline Shear School of Education at SUNY Geneseo where she teaches disability studies courses in Education, Women's Studies, and a writing seminar entitled 'Disability in America.' She investigates the introduction of disability studies in educational settings that range from elementary school classrooms to interdisciplinary coursework in higher education. Her articles have appeared in *Hypatia*, the *National Women's Studies Journal, The International Journal of Inclusive Education, The Society for Disability Studies, Journal of Literary & Cultural Disability Studies, The Journal of Teacher Education, Educational Researcher, Learning Disability Quarterly*, and numerous book chapters. Her book, *Ideology and the Politics of (In)exclusion* has been recognized as one of the earliest collections of critical disability studies scholarship.

Index

For Product Safety Concerns and Information please contact our EU
representative GPSR@taylorandfrancis.com
Taylor & Francis Verlag GmbH, Kaufingerstraße 24, 80331 München, Germany

* 9 7 8 1 1 3 8 0 8 4 9 4 0 *